Issues in Transnational Policing

Globalisation, the wired planet, the global village, these are a few of the terms associated with the social and political changes that are said to describe the world at the beginning of the new millennium. One of the most important institutions of governance has been that of policing, but very little has been written on how the practices of social ordering are affected by the processes of transnationalisation. This book brings together contributions by experts on policing that focus on some of the newly emergent issues connected with these changes:

- the global private security industry
- cross-national networking between police
- the establishment of an international criminal court
- money laundering
- policing cyberspace
- the drug war

Issues in Transnational Policing crosses the boundaries between criminology, international relations and international law to provide a thought-provoking picture of the complex issues surrounding the politics of policing in the future.

James Sheptycki is Lecturer in Sociology, University of Durham.

T0174980

Issues in Transnational Policing

Edited by J. W. E. Sheptycki

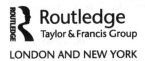

Routledge
Taylor & Francis Group

LONDON AND NEW YORK

First published 2000
by Routledge
2 Park Square, Milton Park, Abingdon, Oxon OX14 4RN

Simultaneously published in the USA and Canada
by Routledge
711 Third Avenue, New York, NY 10017

*Routledge is an imprint of the Taylor & Francis Group,
an informa business*

© 2000 J. W. E. Sheptycki

Typeset in Times by
The Running Head Limited, Cambridge

British Library Cataloguing in Publication Data
A catalogue record for this book is available from the British Library

Library of Congress Cataloging in Publication Data
Issues in transnational policing / edited by J. W. E. Sheptycki.
    p. cm.
Includes bibliographical references and index.
1. Police—International cooperation. I. Sheptycki, J. W. E., 1960–

HV7921.I77 2000
363.2—dc21   00–025484

ISBN 0–415–19260–9 (hbk)
ISBN 0–415–19261–7 (pbk)

For Nana

Contents

viii   *Contents*

Contributors

James Sheptycki is a lecturer in sociology at Durham University. As an undergraduate he studied sociology and international relations at the University of Saskatchewan. He gained a Master of Arts degree from Essex University in the field of political philosophy in 1985. His Ph.D. (London School of Economics 1991) was awarded for research on the policing of domestic violence. His present interest is in bridging the disciplinary divide between international relations, international law and the sociology of policing. He is the Editor of *Policing and Society* and has published in a wide variety of academic journals including *The British Journal of Sociology, The British Journal of Criminology, The International Journal of the Sociology of Law, The International Criminal Justice Review* and *Theoretical Criminology.*

Didier Bigo is Professor of Politics at the Institut d'Etudes Politiques, Paris. His publications include *Police en réseaux: l'experience européenne* (Presses de la Fondation Nationale de Sciences Politiques, 1996). He is also Chief Editor of *Cultures et Conflits.*

Jean-Paul Brodeur is Professor of Criminology at the School of Criminology at the University of Montréal and was formerly the Director of the International Centre for Comparative Criminology there. He is widely published in both English and French. One of his recent publications is *Violence and Racial Prejudice in the Context of Peacekeeping* (Government Services Canada, 1997), which considered the deployment of Canadian forces in Somalia in 1993.

Frank Gregory is Jean Monnet Professor of Politics at the University of Southampton. He has published widely in academic journals on topics relating to international policing and is currently involved in ESRC-funded research on policing organised crime in the former Soviet Union.

Les Johnston is Research Professor at the Institute of Criminal Justice Studies, Portsmouth University. His first book, *The Rebirth of Private Policing* (Routledge, 1992) marked the resurgence of interest in the private security industry in the United Kingdom. His current research interest is in global governance and private forms of security provision.

Peter K. Manning is Professor of Sociology and Psychiatry at Michigan State University. He is the author and editor of over fourteen books and many journal articles. His research concerns embrace the sociology of policing, organisational communication, semiotics and criminology.

Preface

Scholarly interest in policing is relatively recent. As Robert Reiner has explained in numerous articles and books, academic research on policing was virtually non-existent until the 1960s. It was during that decade that it somehow became possible to ask questions about the institutions of social ordering that had long been taken for granted. The result has been a large corpus of work that crosses the whole range of social science and humanistic disciplines from anthropology to political science and socio-legal studies. From William Westley's and Michael Banton's path-breaking work onwards, the study of policing practices has grown steadily, but the contemporary generation of scholars following in the wake of those pioneers of policing research are working in very different circumstances. In the heady days of the 1960s and early 1970s, when academic research on policing was just beginning to gain recognition, its practitioners were likely to bear witness at the sharp end of policing, as the quietude of college and university campuses in many countries erupted into scenes of protest. Such scenes became fewer and farther between in North America and Europe towards the end of the 1980s and, as the century drew to a close, student politics at the universities returned to somnolence. Policing institutions had been the wall against which a generation no longer satisfied with the domestic *status quo* beat their heads, but university campuses are more quiescent these days. In times of great uncertainty politics cautiously cleave to the centre, but this too may change. In the meantime, caught between the gritty but limited pragmatism of criminological 'realism' and the hopeful and non-programmatic utopianism of criminological 'idealism', the study of policing has been reduced to two streams. On the one hand are the scholars interested in policing society and on the other are those interested in policing the police. Some are interested in a synthesis of these two concerns, but this does not change the fact that over the recent past the study of police and policing has, on the whole, been progressively reduced and narrowed to a set of legal and technical concerns despite its earlier evident success in establishing itself as a *bona fide* field of intellectual inquiry.

As the violent twentieth century drew to a close, crime panics and concerns about policing featured prominently in the media, as they had over the preceding decades. What had become different was that policing news was global news. It is not just that on any given day we are more likely to be exposed to images of baton-wielding riot police in far-off lands than we are to such images from close to home. Nor is it just because police-related scandals of one sort or another make good news copy the world over and, hence, course easily through the veins of the international news services and have assured television coverage in any and every jurisdiction. It is also that, in the present period, processes of social change, sometimes referred to as 'globalisation', are changing the way we live our lives in far-reaching ways. As the established patterns of social and political life are re-arranged, the way in which its ordering is achieved also changes. The great varieties of policing institutions that exist are being transformed as a result of these global shifts, with consequences for the discourse of 'due process' and 'crime control'. This has historically provided the key terms for understanding the sociology, politics and legality of policing, but it has been articulated within the parochial confines of the municipality or of the nation-state. Transnational forms of policing are much more in evidence today than they were at the inception of sociological studies of policing and this is symptomatic of a realignment of the state-system that is ongoing. There are a myriad number of transnational practices that impinge on policing in local contexts. In a time of such flux, the narrowing of 'police studies' to a one–two combination (what works in policing – how to make policing accountable) cannot be so easily maintained. It is not that these questions have lost their importance, it is that the circumstances in which such questions are being asked are now quite different from when the field was originally staked out. Then too, because of the wider political and sociological concerns that underpin scholarly interest in police work, the study of transnational policing can be expected to shed considerable light on much bigger questions and so is likely to be of more than particular interest.

The study of policing is being opened up again as a consequence of transnationalisation. The breadth of disciplinary concerns that informed the field in its initial phase are again being drafted in. This book is an attempt at addressing some of the salient issues that arise from concerns about transnationalisation. It seeks to add to the stock of ideas that animate the study of policing. A second concern, to show how policing shapes the contours of the evolving transnational-state-system, is equally important. My background in international relations, a foundation laid as an undergraduate student at the University of Saskatchewan in Canada, and my academic apprenticeship in the study of policing, gained as a Ph.D. student at the London School of Economics, are thus brought into happy coincidence. The result, I hope, is a new set of research questions that will capture the interest of readers across the world who work in any and all of the social sciences and humanistic disciplines.

I owe a debt of gratitude to many people who have helped me to take these ideas forward or who have simply offered their quiet but sustaining interest. At the risk of causing offence by omission, I wish to thank: Robert Reiner, Richard Ericson, Philip Stenning, Clifford Shearing, Stan Cohen, David Bayley, Malcolm Anderson, Neil Walker, William Gilmore, Peter Cullen, Charles Raab, Cyrille Fijnaut, Lode van Outrive, 'Tank' Waddington, Clive Emsley, Mike Maguire, Monica den Boer, Dick Hobbs, Mike Levi, Mike Brogden, David Downes, Paul Rock, Gary Marx, Ben Bowling, Janet Chan, Ian Loader, Mathieu Deflem, Monique Marks, Andrew Goldsmith, Dawn Bennet, Valsamis Mitsilegas, Pat O'Malley, Peter Andreas, David Wall, David Garland, Andrew Crawford, Kevin Haggerty, Karim Murji, Eugene McLaughlin, Kevin Stenson, Trevor Jones, Willem De Lint, Paddy Rawlinson, Detlef Nogala, Christine Boch, Claude Journés, Rob and Marja Witte, Anne Flaveau, Marleena Easton, Janne Flyghed, Patrick Doelle, 'Squire T', Machiel Roerink, Frank Gallagher, Colin Philips, Paul Swallow, Johan Denolf, and Peter Stelfox. All of them have helped me to sustain this research interest in one way or another and I am most grateful to them. I am also extremely grateful to the other contributors to this volume. Lastly, I must thank my family and friends who have helped along the way. Without their support and forbearance this work could not have been completed.

J. W. E. Sheptycki
University of Durham

Introduction

James Sheptycki

What is transnational policing? The answer to this question is not easy to find, not least because the traditional boundaries between various disciplines (criminology, international relations, international law and the like) have been drawn in such a way that such an issue has not been raised. This volume aims to begin answering the question and it does so in such a way that it will kindle the interest of students and researchers who are only beginning their careers. The intention is to open up a field of inquiry and consequently the book does not offer an encyclopaedic compendium of work done in the area. The fact is that what I refer to as 'transnational policing' is a recent conceptual innovation and the phenomena to which it refers have not been comprehensively researched. It is my contention that transnational policing, like a host of other transnational phenomena, will be a crucial concern in the coming years as social life is increasingly lived beyond the parochial confines of traditional ways of living. For those who share my view, the contributions herein are likely to be of great interest.

The idea for this volume was to bring together some contributions by colleagues and friends whose interest in the study of social control on the global stage had also been piqued early on. I approached a number of people with the idea for an edited collection that would both spark the interests of students and carve out a research problematic. The resulting volume may well raise as many questions as it answers, but it should also take the process of refining the conceptual apparatus necessary to this specific intellectual inquiry quite a good distance. Before overviewing the contributions to the volume it is necessary to spend some time discussing the basic concepts, viz.: the notions of 'transnational' and of 'policing'. On these two words the project rides and if their meaning is simply obvious then the whole project ends where it starts. It is my view that the terms are not at all self-evident and students who wish to tackle the vexing issues of 'transnational organised crime', 'human smuggling', 'sex tourism', 'air rage' and similar crime panics that currently feature so prominently in various news media, or those who wish to understand the political and legal nuances of the putative 'global order' of the twenty-first century generally, would do well to focus on precisely these terms.

The task of this introductory chapter is threefold. Firstly, I will overview some of the more salient literature regarding transnational-isation and associated terms. The second, and in my view more com-plicated, task is to put forward some definitions and a typology for understanding policing. Lastly, I shall overview the various contribu-tions to the volume and show how a research problematic is slowly being built up in the interstices of traditional academic modes of inquiry. A paradigm, as Kuhn observed, does not so much consist in a defined set of answers, but rather consists in the set of questions conventionally asked. By establishing a set of analytical tools, suggest-ing pertinent questions and indicating ways in which we might go about answering them, *Issues in Transnational Policing* is an attempt to position a new paradigm in social research. If you are interested in questions regarding the social and political order of the transnational era, then read on.

Defining the transnational

It was at the beginning of the 1970s that the multinational firm be-came an object of public concern in what was termed, euphemistically, the 'developed world'. As one author put it: 'the time has come for governments everywhere to decide what to do about the great multi-national companies that have grown up in the last twenty-five years' (Tugendhat 1971: 1). Actually, the concerns about the relative auto-nomy of multinational behemoths from direct and uncompromised control by national governments had been raised among experts some-what earlier. For example, the Royal Institute of International Affairs at Chatham House hosted two private conferences in 1968 and 1970 on the problems arising from the growth of these institutions. On the other side of the Atlantic, Robert Keohan and Joseph Nye were also beginning to think about international relations in a way that de-parted from the entrenched 'state centred' approach that characterised American 'realist' foreign policy thinking (Keohane and Nye 1972/ 1981: vii). As they understood it, there was an important job to do in mapping the patterns of interaction between a variety of international organisations, not least of which were the multinationals. These con-cerns came to public attention in an explosive manner during the oil crisis of 1974. It was not just that the OPEC countries could bring Europe and North America to their knees by shutting off oil exports – it was during that crisis that it was suddenly brought to everyone's attention what fantastic profits the multinational oil companies had been making since 1945. Conspiracy theories about the role of the 'Seven Sisters' abounded and in that moment, what John Burton (1972) called the 'billiard ball model' of international relations, wherein relations between sovereign nation-states are considered the proper, indeed only, focus of international relations, was made contestable.

The nation-state is understood here in standard Weberian terms, as an institution that upholds the right of binding rule-making over a defined territory by reason of a monopoly of the legitimate use of coercive force (Jessop 1982). Such states are understood to comprise an international order or 'state-system', and this system is, perhaps, the prime accomplishment of modernity (Tilley 1975). The nation-state cannot be understood as an entity existing by itself, but only as part of a larger system. As Talcott Parsons (1971) observed, three nations, England, France and Holland 'were the spearhead of early modernity' (p. 54). The emergence of these three entities commenced a period of 'state-making' whereby an earlier form of political sovereignty, characterised as the King-state (Giddens 1985; Anderson 1996) was gradually supplanted. Charles Tilley and like-minded intellectuals have traced the process whereby Europe was reduced from some 500 more or less independent political units in 1500 to twenty-odd states by 1900. Such an attenuated historical process was inevitably uneven, proceeding from numerous causes under various conditions, and therefore cannot be reduced to a simple linear schema. Suffice it to say that by the dawn of the twentieth century the state-system was poised to expand yet further and over the course of that century remap the globe. Tilley ended his own account of this process in an open-ended manner, noting that 'at the same time as the state system absorbs the entire world, the individual state may be losing part of its significance' (1975: 638). He speculated about the devolution of the power of the nation-state 'both upward and downward' and suggested that this configuration of power was in part determined by the nature of the markets, capital, communications capabilities and productive capacities of the era in which such states emerged (ibid.). As the nature of markets change and the transnational flow of capital broadens, deepens and increases in speed; as the technical capacity for communications within productive systems and other social institutions is enhanced; in short, as the processes of transnationalisation unfold, the very bases for the emergence and sustenance of the nation-state-system alter. And yet

4 *James Sheptycki*

the vocabulary of international relations continues to dominate our thinking about world politics (Ruggie 1993). The billiard ball model that Burton criticised remains a feature of our thinking and international relations are still often conceived as pertaining only to relations between sovereign nation-states.

One attempt to overcome the limitations of the vocabulary of international relations was to be found in the work of Ramon Aron who, in the mid-1960s, tried to introduce the concept of 'transnational society' into that body of theory (Aron 1966). For him, transnational relations consisted of commercial interchanges, the migration of persons and ideas and the practices of non-state organisations that transgressed state-defined frontiers. However, in examining social formations as various as those of Europe just prior to World War I and fifth-century BC Greece, he came to the conclusion that, even where transnational relations and processes are robust, there is a relative autonomy of the interstate order and further suggested that this relative autonomy meant that relations between states *per se* remained the foundation for understanding world politics. In other words, that early shift in vocabulary was not enough to challenge the main assumptions of international relations theory; in the mid 1960s the Cold War was hot and Dr Henry Kissinger was about to launch a secret war in Cambodia which had all the logic of *Machtpolitik*, a principal variant of realist international relations theory (Shawcross 1979). The contemporary landscape simply obscured the insights that this shift in vocabulary might have yielded.

Somewhat later, Robert Keohane and Joseph Nye (1971/1981) seized upon the idea of transnational society and sought to develop it further. According to them transnational relations were, in fact, nothing new. Neither did they want to argue that transnational relations had entirely superseded relations between states on the world stage. In expressing these views they did not differ significantly from Aron's position. However, they went on to argue that a whole variety of transnational relations affect interstate politics in profound ways. As they put it, transnational processes 'affect interstate politics by altering the choices open to statesmen and the costs that must be borne for adopting various course of action' (pp. 374–5). Significantly, they pointed out that over the bulk of recorded history human beings have been organised for political purposes on bases other than those subsumed under the concept of 'state' and 'nation-state'. By taking a wider historical perspective, the naturalness of the assumptions of realist international relations theory looked less engaging. Still, at the height of the Cold War, it was impractical to argue that state actors did not hold centre stage, even if other institutions were recognised as playing an important part in world politics.

The year 1989 was thus an extremely important marker. The abrupt end of the Cold War brought new challenges to thinking about international politics. Then, too, the processes illuminated only a decade earlier were much more apparent. As John Gerard Ruggie (1993) noted, there had been a remarkable growth in transnational micro-economic links since World War II. He pointed to 'the markets and production facilities that are designated by the awkward term "offshore" – as though they existed in some ethereal space waiting to be reconceived by an economic equivalent of relativity theory' (p. 141). Ethereal it might seem, but it is in the offshore arena that sourcing, production and marketing can be organised within 'global factories'; the work of lawyers and accountants can be orchestrated in 'global offices'; and scientific research can be structured in the 'global lab'. Crucially, real-time transnational information flows are the raw material of all three. Further, 'financial transactions take place in various "Euro" facilities, which may be *housed* in Tokyo, New York and European financial centres but which are considered to exist in an extranational realm' (ibid., emphasis in original). The offshore banking system is an important facet of the transnational realm and the existence of havens for capital which are beyond the control of nation-states has raised important new questions, not least for criminology (see chapter five). To paraphrase Eric Hobsbawm (1994), in the crisis years since 1973 the international economy has become 'uncontrollable' resulting in 'an era in which the national state has lost its powers'. The enormous and perhaps even incalculable wealth hidden in offshore banks is testimony to the de-centring of the state in the transnational age.

Then too, the development of the power of transnational capital must be seen as operating in conjunction with a simultaneous process engendered by the success of neo-liberal politics. The agenda set by neo-liberalism holds that, in order for specific regions or states to remain competitive within the global market-place, the cost of governance has to be reduced (Pratt 1999). The adoption of the strategy of privatisation, by no means universal in the 'developed world' but nevertheless pervasive and ongoing, has affected a whole range of services provided by the state. The catalogue extends beyond the privatisation of state-owned utilities (such as rail, power and water systems) to include health, education and other types of social welfare provision including, in some places, parts of the criminal justice system. A number of states which have been until quite recently structured along Keynesian lines have been significantly 'pared back'. Thus it can be argued that the erosion of the nation-state is happening both 'from above' and 'from below' (Sheptycki 1998a).

There is a need to exercise some caution here. It would be a mistake to take these observations too far. To argue that transnationalisation has fundamentally altered the conditions of the state-system is not the same as arguing that states are no longer important institutions in global politics. Fred Halliday (1994) has made this point, perhaps somewhat too stridently. He says of Keohane's later work that it both overstated the degree of decline of the state's influence in the world and inflated the role of the supposedly successor transnational institutions. Further, according to Halliday, Keohane failed to recognise the ways in which US military predominance and leadership, something that has continued after the Cold War, had economic and other 'seigniorial benefits' (p. 30). This overstates Keohane's position. According to him, 'understanding the general principles of state actions and the practices of governments is a necessary basis for attempts to refine theory or to extend the analysis to non-state actors'. Further, 'approaches using new concepts may be able to supplement, enrich or extend a basic theory of state action, but they cannot substitute for it' (Keohane 1989: 35). We can cut through this muddle by making a clear distinction between 'transnationalisation' and 'globalisation'. The former attempts to understand action on the global stage by reference to state action as it is conditioned by non-state factors and processes in world politics. The latter overstates the case, characterising the newly emergent world order as one where states have been disempowered and wholly subordinated to the power of transnational capital.

Transnational relations, and attendant concepts, also direct our attention to another important facet of world politics. Not only are non-state actors important, in some of the literature there is an attempt to understand the influence of sub-state actors. By sub-state actors we mean individuals or institutions who form part of the machinery of state but who do not themselves represent the sovereign power of the state in the transnational domain. To say that sub-state actors are of some significance in the transnational-state-system is more than the assertion of Charles Beard's classic admonishment that 'foreign policy is a phase of domestic policy'. It is a corrective to Kenneth Waltz's plausible assertion that 'it is not possible to understand world politics simply by looking inside of states' (Waltz 1979: 65). Halliday (1994) reminds us that while we cannot understand international relations 'simply by looking inside states', this is 'quite different from arguing that the internal processes of states can be excluded altogether from a theorisation of international relations' (p. 36). The move from saying that international relations cannot be studied 'simply' by looking at the internal working of states to saying the internal workings can be ignored is invalid. It is particularly so when we see sub-state actors acting in important ways in the transnational arena. This latter point becomes readily apparent when we consider the role that various public police agencies have played in this realm. While it might be true to say that the public police are representatives of the state's sovereign authority within the territory of a given state, they are not themselves sovereign representatives in the transnational sphere (see the chapters by Brodeur and Bigo in this volume).

Transnationalisation summary

From the above discussion it should be clear that transnational relations are made up of a wide variety of transnational practices. This view is in contrast to that of international relations which focuses on the practices of sovereign states, the prime – although by no means only – examples of which are war and conquest (Waltz 1959). Transnational relations and practices are long-standing, indeed there is a sense in which such interactions pre-date the nation-state system itself. Over the course of the nineteenth and early to mid-twentieth centuries, international relations have dominated our conception of world politics, but in the contemporary period the balance has shifted and, in the transnational era, the state is no longer centre stage. Indeed, as the multiple processes of transnationalisation unfold, the world stage has become crowded with actors, many of whom are relatively autonomous from the state-system and often do not act in the interests of states. Then, too, because of these processes, the actions of sub-state actors seem more important to understand than they once did. To use this vocabulary is to eschew the radical globalisation thesis, wherein states are visualised as the neutered instruments of an outmoded type of social power. At the same time, it suggests that to understand world politics and social ordering in the contemporary period is to abandon the realist assumptions of international relations that illuminate only the actions of the diplomats, soldiers and other highly decorated representatives of the sovereign power of the state, and to look at the actions of a wide variety of other actors as well. In short we no longer study the nation-state system, but rather look at the transnational-state-system. The role that policing plays in the transnational-state-system is a crucial one. Thus, it is necessary to unpack what we mean by that term.

Defining policing

The presiding definition of 'police' was fixed as a term of discourse, at least in the sociological literature, with the publication of Egon Bittner's *The Functions of Police in Modern Society* (1970). In that book Bittner focused attention on the formation of the modern police which, according to him, formed 'the last basic building block of modern executive government' (p. 15). He noted that the establishment of governance in this period was characterised by a 'progressive avoidance of force ... evident in changes in the administration of justice' (p. 18). In a remarkable anticipation of Norbert Elias's 'civilising process' thesis, Bittner observed that there was, over the course of the nineteenth century, a general move away from political authority based purely on threats or the exercise of physical force towards one based on voluntary performances of the governed. This is, according to Bittner's view, part of a general cultural shift and he cites several examples to support this, one of which is the gradual disappearance of weaponry as an accoutrement of male attire. He then argues that 'it would seem to be exceedingly unlikely that the idea of modern police could have arisen in any other cultural context' (p. 21). Since the complete pacification of society, the elimination of all violence and the consummation of 'Civilisation' are ultimately not achievable, there is a necessity to invest an institution with the power to use coercion in order to ensure social order with a minimum of violence. That institution is the 'public police' and its creation follows the logic of the civilising process (and is embedded in the state-making process sketched in the previous section). To paraphrase Bittner, it is necessary to ensure that 'the exercise of provoked force required to meet illegitimate attacks' is held to the 'minimum consistent with social order'. In order to do that, 'special forms of authorisation' in the conduct of coercion are required and that is done through the institution of a police force.

It is possible to take issue with the 'civilisation thesis', as Zygmunt Bauman (1989) has done. In a century that has produced two world wars, a host of smaller (but no less bloody) conflicts and numerous attempts at genocide, assertions regarding the gradual elimination of violence appear rather weak. Bittner recognised that he was painting a 'one sided exaggeration', and he doubtless could formulate a reply. Certainly others who pursue the general tenets of the 'civilisation thesis' have a rejoinder to Bauman, and this might be taken to reside in the rise of human rights discourse in the post-1945 period (cf. Cohen 1994). However, this broad debate need not concern us here. What does concern us is a particular limitation on our understanding of policing that emerges from Bittner's sociology. He focused almost exclusively on the activities of uniformed patrol officers. While it is certainly important to cultivate an understanding of the uniformed public police as the repositories of the state's monopoly of coercive force in the maintenance of the internal social order of the state's territory, it is misguided to think that understanding policing can be reduced to understanding the activities of uniformed patrol officers. There is much more to policing than 'cops on the beat'.

Jean-Paul Brodeur introduced an important distinction between 'high' and 'low' policing into the lexicon of the sociology of policing (Brodeur 1983). Political police, 'high police' in Brodeur's terms, are a crucial aspect of policing, both historically and contemporaneously. Yet, as Richard Thurlow (1994) has observed, 'this is a subject which government would prefer academics and others should ignore' (p. 1). Indeed, by focusing so intently on the tasks of uniformed patrol and, to a somewhat lesser extent, on the work of criminal investigations police, much of the social scientific literature on the topic does precisely that. Discussions of 'police accountability', for example, invariably limit the target to the political accountability of municipal policing. This limitation is becoming increasingly untenable as 'high policing' agencies, including the CIA in America, MI5 and the British Special Branch in Britain, and a host of others, are drafted in to engage with 'organised crime' and other 'serious crime'. Bringing the 'high police' function back into the discussion is difficult because it is so often obscured by the very terminology used to describe it. Thus Frank Donner (1980) has noted that our terms for explaining political policing ('internal security', 'national security', 'intelligence gathering', etc.) have become so euphemistic that 'their meaning has been ravaged, reduced to disembodied buzz words' (p. xv). Yet clearly this form of policing is a crucial element in the maintenance of social order, because it attends to those policing tasks that aim to secure the integrity of the state itself and, in the contemporary period, because 'high police' now have an active and acknowledged role in controlling 'ordinary law crime' (for an historical excursion into these issues see Mazower 1997). The distinction between 'high' and 'low' policing brings an added degree of complexity to our understanding. Connectedly, Gary Marx (1980) has also noted that the dominant orientation in the sociological literature on policing stresses the role of uniformed police and of criminal investigation, especially as it is mobilised by citizen requests. This, he says, is entirely in keeping with democratic conceptions of the right and proper role of governance in modern societies, but it is increasingly at odds with the reality of police work, a growing proportion of which has been given over to 'proactive' and 'undercover' police. Marx ploughed a lonely furrow until quite recently. However, because of the steady growth in such police operations on a world-wide basis and especially in the context of the 'war on drugs', this aspect of police work has slowly come into focus. Now the term 'undercover policing' and ones associated with it have assumed a prominence in the litera-ture roughly commensurate with their importance in policing practice (Fijnaut and Marx 1995).

Bittner confined the study of policing in another way which is no longer tenable. It was during the late 1970s in the United States that some researchers began to notice the prevalence of profit-oriented police services. Steven Spitzer and Andrew Scull (1977) cited statistics showing that roughly two out of every three police officers in the USA were actually on private payrolls. According to them, the 'big four' of the 'rent-a-cop' industry had revenues in excess of US $640 million per annum. Somewhat later, in Canada, Philip Stenning and Clifford Shear-ing noted a 'quiet revolution' that had undermined the centrality of state-centred policing (Stenning and Shearing 1980). In the United Kingdom, Nigel South argued that 'the post-war expansion of the private security sector has revolutionary implications for the nature of modern social control and the policing of society . . . such a significant increase in resort to private arrangements for ensuring security has fundamentally changed society's division of policing labour' (p. 150). Clearly an adequate understanding of policing requires us to examine not only state forms; our definition must encompass private policing as well. There is, by now, a broad and growing literature on private policing (see Jones and Newburn 1998), but much of it ignores the transnational aspects of the business (Johnston, this volume).

There is another definition worth considering when we try to pro-vide a set of terms for grasping the practices of policing. Police are agents who aim to ensure a modicum of 'social order' and they do so by performing something called 'social control'. But what does this entail? A useful distinction has been made: conceptualising police work between 'securing territory' and controlling 'suspect populations' (Ericson and Carriere 1994; Ericson 1994). This distinction might be considered more analytic than practical since there is a sense in which the securing of territory requires that the large majority of its popula-tion is successfully brought under a system of formal social control. Conversely, in order for a population to be brought under a system of formal social control, the territory on which that population resides must also be secure. The practice of 'peace enforcement' in the former Yugoslavia, in parts of Africa and elsewhere makes this abundantly

Table 1 A typology of policing

	Police work aimed at securing territory		Police work aimed at securing populations	
	Private forms	*Public forms*	*Private forms*	*Public forms*
High policing	Corporate security guards	Guardians of the state apparatus	Corporate security specialists	State security and the Secret Service
Low policing	Private security guards	Uniformed patrol officers	Private eyes	Police detectives

clear. Yet, the practical intertwining of these aspects of police work does not preclude our making the analytical distinction. Indeed, although the surveillance of suspect populations is contingent on the mastery of territory and vice versa, there are practical differences that need to be understood. Some of these differences will become more clear in a moment.

The terminology for understanding the practices of policing is thus contained within three conceptual distinctions: between 'high' and 'low' policing; between public and private forms of policing; and between policing activity aimed at securing territory or controlling populations. The divisions thus described can be laid out, as in the typology in Table 1.

The cells of this table are worthy of disquisition at length. All that can be undertaken here is an overview; the result is suggestive and illustrative, rather than definitive and encyclopaedic.

1 Corporate security guards. This form of policing practice is likely to be of increasing interest in the research literature although there is little systematic work on it to date. Nevertheless, in the office environment of the private corporate world there has arisen a heightened perception about the problems associated with 'industrial espionage'. The provision of access control and monitoring systems to secure office buildings, or parts of office buildings, is an expression of the need to control corporate territory. Research and development facilities are especially likely to be well guarded. Access to secure sites in the corporate milieu is controlled by a variety of technical devices which are familiar enough. CCTV systems, smart

card systems, entry and access systems, and systems to control the territory of 'cyberspace' within the computers of large multinational corporations, are just a few examples of the performance of the high policing function on corporate territory. How do physical guards protect intangible property rights (patents and copyrights)?

2 Guardians of the state apparatus. This is more familiar ground, even if it has been ignored in virtually all studies of policing. Here we are concerned with the security of the buildings of state and other aspects of the territorial integrity of the state. A number of terrorist attacks in the USA in the recent period have awakened an interest in these aspects of the policing role, but here again, the sociology of policing literature is largely inadequate. Some of the technological aspects are familiar enough and there are some instances where private companies have won contracts to secure buildings housing elements of the state bureaucracy. The interplay between the public and private spheres is unclear. What does it mean when a large multinational security firm wins a contract to provide security to government buildings (for example, The Pentagon)?

3/4 Corporate security specialists. State security and the secret service. There is a fascinating interplay between the public and private domain practices of the surveillance of suspect populations in the high policing functions which makes the analytical distinction all the more crucial. There is an interest in keeping employees working within secure institutional sites, in both the state and private sectors, under surveillance. Having secured the space or territory where 'classified' activity takes place (cells 1 and 2), police systems are concerned to maintain surveillance over the activities of those who have right of entry to such institutional enclaves. One particular concern is obviously the monitoring of employee activity in cyberspace, but surveillance of both civilian workers working for private corporations and of state employees working within the state apparatus (that is protecting against either industrial or political espionage) may also involve keeping these special populations under surveillance after office hours and well away from the place of work (see Manning, this volume). High policing in this mode may also include keeping up surveillance of, on the one hand, business competitors, and on the other hand, the personnel working on behalf of other political entities. Espionage on behalf of the state may blur into espionage on behalf of private corporations. A report published by the European Parliament (http://www.europarl.eu.int/dg4/stoa/en/publi/166499/), citing an article in the *Sunday Times* (11 May 1998), notes a number of instances where the US National Security Agency (NSA) was purported to have passed on industrial secrets to US companies, giving them a competitive economic advantage. One such allegation suggests that Thompson-CSF, a French electronics company, lost a $1.4 billion deal to supply Brazil with a radar system because the NSA intercepted details of the negotiations and passed them on to US company Raytheon, which subsequently won the contract. Another such claim was that Airbus Industrie lost a contract worth $1 billion to Boeing and McDonnell Douglas because information was intercepted and passed on by the NSA. Yet a third instance of this blurring is the case of a German company, Enercon, which lost its ability to patent a new form of wind-generating technology to an American competitor, Kenetech, after the NSA tapped the telephone and computer links between Enercon's research lab and its production facility and subsequently passed on detailed plans of the invention to Kenetech. Details of this latter case emerged when a former NSA employee appeared on German television.

High policing on behalf of the state is especially concerned with 'subversion', that is, activity thought to compromise the security of the state. This is a well researched area (Donner 1980; Lustgarten and Leigh 1994; Whitaker and Marcuse 1994). What is, as yet, under-researched is the extent to which private forms of policing are involved in these activities. Nor do we know much about the ways in which these two spheres interact. Lastly, there are a set of issues emergent in the contemporary period surrounding the 'ecological movement' and so-called 'eco-terrorism'. Some industries, for example cosmetics and pharmaceuticals, have been the target of such actions on the grounds that they undertake experiments on live animals. Responsibility for policing eco-terrorism has been taken up by public police agencies and, in the United Kingdom, Special Branch has been most involved in this activity.

5   Private security guards. The 'Pinkerton Man', strolling the shopping mall and preserving an atmosphere conducive to the social order of consumption, or the security services associated with the 'gated community' have a well established place in the research literature on policing. Private guards secure the territory for very localised, not to say parochial, domains, and yet they are likely to be employed by multinational firms (Johnston, this volume). In the contemporary period privatised forms of social control are changing the shape of urban space in profound ways (Davis 1992), and this is happening globally (Sheptycki 1997), but it is not certain

that private security is actually eroding, eclipsing or eliding public forms of policing (Jones and Newburn 1998; Yoshida 1999). But there are other domains where private security providers are very active and yet remain under-researched: production facilities in 'destabilised' regions such as Colombia or Russia, resource extraction sites in similar regions, corporate executives who travel globally, all require security services and intelligence – often euphemistically referred to as 'risk management' – which is procured from privately owned companies or undertaken by in-house security departments.

6   Uniformed patrol officers. The patrol officer on 'skid row' is a dominant image in the sociology of policing literature. Indeed, Bittner may appear to have exhausted the analytic potential of this role. However, the routines of public policing have been reconfigured by ongoing technological revolution which knows no national boundaries. For example, Geographic Information Systems and the Compstat System, together with a range of technical devices that enhance the police's coercive capacities, have changed the way public police patrol is undertaken. Technology transfer is one of the main vehicles for the transnationalisation of policing (Sheptycki 1998b). The activities of public police in securing territory are affected in complex ways by the processes of transnationalisation. To cite but one, perhaps trivial, example: in the transnational age the activities of uniformed patrol officers have been extended to removing the perpetrators of 'air rage' from grounded aircraft. Also, the activities of border police, who aim to protect the territorial integrity of states from incursions of illegal immigrants and smugglers, have achieved a new prominence in the contemporary period. These changes mean that the academic literature on policing will, of necessity, maintain a central concern with the work of public police.

7   Private eyes. The fictional image of Philip Marlowe looms large here, but private detectives are busy with much less glamorous business. Investigating insurance fraud is probably the largest element of policing work that comes under this heading. Then, too, corporate entities encounter risks of many sorts and some of them are amenable to the arts of private detectives. Kidnappings of corporate executives working overseas, product contamination, extortion and asset recovery are just a few examples of the roles which private security experts have assumed in policing on behalf of corporate order. This type of police work has a very low profile in the academic literature.

8 Police detectives. The 'undercover cop', long the province of crime
   fiction and, until relatively recently, virtually ignored in the academic literature on policing, will continue to engage the attention
   of social science researchers. Indeed, there are indications that
   'intelligence-led policing' has become the new paradigm for the
   public police (Sheptycki 2000), but the spread of this model is
   uneven and there is a need to chart its development. As policing
   becomes more proactive and less reactive, as it becomes more
   interested in forms of risk assessment for specific individuals within
   general categories of suspect population, and as forms of serious
   and organised crime come to take priority within policing policy,
   this type of role will grow. The introduction of various 'high police'
   agencies into this domain sets up new patterns of interaction which
   have yet to be fully examined. The technical developments that
   enable these shifts in emphasis are transnational, as are the crime
   panics that fuel them.

Policing summary

The above discussion has shown that policing can be understood by
reference to three principal conceptual sub-divisions: between the 'high'
and 'low' policing functions; between 'private' and 'public' police provision; and between the policing of 'suspect populations' and the policing to control a given territory. These conceptual distinctions yield
an eightfold typology, as shown in Table 1. Although consideration
of the conceptual grid that these analytic distinctions establish has
been partial here, enough has been said to establish that policing is
much more than 'stout men in blue coats' (Reiner 1988). Examination
of this typology has also given some partial indication of how the
processes of transnationalisation impact on the various categories of
policing. Academic inquiry into the social and political practices
of policing will thus, of necessity, move along a broad front. A word
of caution needs to be injected here. A typology of the sort laid out in
the previous section might serve to create the appearance that each cell
somehow carries equal weight. It therefore must be acknowledged at
the outset that each of these types of police function is separate and
distinct, even as these policing roles are intertwined in complex ways
in the practical day-to-day reality of securing social order. It is not the
case, for example, that we can say that the work of corporate private
security is more or less central to social ordering than is the work of
the public police. Neither is simple recourse to tabulating the number
of personnel in these two spheres, or their financial implications, or

the number of crimes cleared up, or losses prevented, or the amount of assets recovered, or criminal assets seized, or criminal groups detected or disrupted likely to provide a complete answer. We need to ask these sorts of questions, of course, and to give answers to them, but in so doing it is important not to lose sight of the broader field. For too long academic inquiry into the activities that comprise policing has been content with a myopic vision. In the transnational era we increasingly live our lives in the transnational domain and so it is as important to keep our eyes on the horizon as it is to watch where our feet are stepping.

What remains to be done in this introductory chapter is to overview the contributions. The contributing authors were invited to write on topics that interested them according to analytical preferences they chose themselves. The phenomena that underwrite the research problematic around transnational policing mean that inquiry tends towards convergence even without the hegemony of an established research paradigm.

The contributions

Les Johnston's chapter has many obvious points of connection with the discussion pursued in this Introduction. He lays bare the transnational aspects of private security provision. Here Johnston is concerned to map the contours of the global security market, to illuminate the practices that animate it, to address questions about social ordering and governance that arise from the success of neo-liberalism and, in the final analysis, to raise the issue of commercial security and its implications for justice and governance. In chapter two, Jean-Paul Brodeur uses two case studies of transnational police investigations to show how the local (i.e. national) politics of policing are refracted in surprising and unpredictable ways in the transnational realm. He raises questions about how due process of law can be maintained in transnational investigations and shows some ways in which police accountability issues become fraught when the work becomes transnational in scope. In chapter three Didier Bigo looks at the developing network of police liaison officers in Europe. He is especially interested to chart the interconnections between the police, state security, the military, customs and other police-type agents as this growing network struggles to maintain the boundaries of the new European Security Field. The liaison officer in Europe (indeed globally) is the conduit for the exchange of information on suspect populations between national police systems and these networks are well developed. Bigo offers one of the most comprehensive views of this type of police work available. In so doing he observes that the territorial state may cease to be the quintessential form of governance. According to him, as the logic of domination comes to cross national boundaries freely, all the while developing new disciplinary networks, control bureaucracies might then be freed from the juridical limits set by frontiers, which has fundamental implications for the character of governance. Frank Gregory analyses the ways in which particular forms of criminality become matters of international concern which highlights the political processes that underlie the formation of international-criminal law institutions. The creation of transnational criminal law regimes, such as that against piracy and slavery in the nineteenth century and against drug markets in the twentieth are political and moral projects. Gregory examines some of the political and practical issues that arise from the attempt to create transnational control efforts looking in particular at the faltering efforts to create an International Criminal Court and the ways in which the United Nations and the European Union have sought to circumscribe the transnationalisation of certain aspects of social control. The difficulties of establishing a criminal court with universal jurisdiction over a range of transnational crimes, and the corollary of this – that transnational law enforcement takes place within a fragmented legal frame – echo the analysis pursued by both Didier Bigo and Jean-Paul Brodeur. Seen in this light, the discussion in chapter five follows quite naturally. In that chapter I overview the developing transnational effort to control money laundering and the offshore banking world generally. Examination of efforts to control the circuits of transnational finance is set against the 'hollowing out of the state' hypothesis and alternative explanations are explored. The emerging character of global governance can be glimpsed in the processes that have been built up for controlling 'dirty money'. One important point that this chapter establishes is that transnational policing in a fragmented legal setting creates problems for and of law enforcement. This relates again to the emergent character of transnational governance, but the aim of the analysis cannot be so neatly pre-scripted. In the penultimate chapter Peter Manning takes a look at the policing of 'new social spaces'. In a wide-ranging consideration of issues that emerge in the context of a 'wired planet', Manning gives a likely indication of how policing in the twenty-first century might be expected to shift. In doing so he draws particular attention to the fact that social life is increasingly being negotiated through mediated communications, that 'information' and 'knowledge' gain in importance as they are reconstituted as private property and that there are important political and economic consequences that flow from these shifts which affect the way we need to think about control culture. He reminds readers that the processes of social control work as much analogically and metaphorically as they do literally, and thus the representations of transnational crime are of central importance. But in order to understand the images that comprise the pantheon of transnational folk devilry, we must first consider the apparatus of social control that helps to create those images.

The final chapter addresses the paradigm example of transnational policing in the twentieth century, viz: the drug war. It provides a synoptic history of the pursuit of an international drug prohibition regime and examines some of the general lessons that this might offer for our understanding of transnational policing. Central to this analysis is the idea that world-wide drug prohibition can only be properly understood in the context of the evolving transnational state system over the course of the century. International drug prohibition is the flag-ship of the transnational police enterprise and, hence, has assumed centrality in the preoccupations of global governance.

This volume is an attempt to bring the great variety of institutions that pursue the transnational police mission into focus. It is a partial and incomplete picture, to be sure. But I think that it shows clearly that there has been a good deal of solid intellectual work already done and which will no doubt be drawn upon as further explorations of policing in the transnational realm are undertaken.

References

Anderson, M. (1996) *Frontiers: Territory and State Formation in the Modern World*, Cambridge: Polity Press.
Aron, R. (1966) *Peace and War: A Theory of International Relations*, translated by R. Howard and A. Baker Fox, Garden City NY: Doubleday and Co.
Bauman, Z. (1989) *Modernity and the Holocaust*, Ithaca NY: Cornell University Press.
Bittner, E. (1970) *The Functions of Police in Modern Society*, Chevy Chase MD: National Institute of Mental Health.
Brodeur, J.-P. (1983) 'High Policing and Low Policing: Remarks about the Policing of Political Activities' *Social Problems*, Vol. 30, No. 5, pp. 507–20.
Burton, J. (1972) *World Society*, Cambridge: Cambridge University Press.
Cohen, S. (1994) 'Social Control and the Politics of Reconstruction', in D. Nelken (ed.), *The Futures of Criminology*, London: Sage.

Davis, M. (1992) *City of Quartz: Excavating the Future in Los Angeles*, London: Vintage.

Donner, F. H. (1980) *The Age of Surveillance: The Aims and Methods of America's Political Intelligence System*, New York: Alfred A. Knopf.

Ericson, R. V. (1994) 'The Division of Expert Knowledge in Policing and Security', *British Journal of Sociology*, Vol. 45, No. 2, pp. 149–76.

Ericson, R. V. and Carriere, K. (1994) 'The Fragmentation of Criminology', in D. Nelken (ed.), *The Futures of Criminology*, London: Sage.

Fijnaut, C. and Marx, G. (1995) *Undercover: Police Surveillance in Comparative Perspective*, The Hague: Kluwer.

Giddens, A. (1985) *A Contemporary Critique of Historical Materialism*, Vol. 2, *The Nation-State and Violence*, Cambridge: Polity Press.

Halliday, F. (1994) *Rethinking International Relations*, Vancouver: University of British Colombia Press.

Hobsbawm, E. (1994) *The Age of Extremes: The Short Twentieth Century*, London: Michael Joseph.

Jessop, B. (1982) *The Capitalist State*, Oxford: Martin Robertson.

Jones, T. and Newburn, T. (1998) *Private Security and Public Policing*, Oxford: Clarendon Press.

Keohane, R. (1989) *International Institutions and State Power*, Boulder CO: Westview Press.

Keohane, R. and Nye, J. (1972/1981) *Transnational Relations and World Politics*, Cambridge MA: Harvard University Press.

Lustgarten, L. and Leigh, I. (1994) *In from the Cold: National Security and Parliamentary Democracy*, Oxford: Clarendon Press.

Marx, G. T. (1980) 'The New Police Undercover Work', *Urban Life*, Vol. 8, No. 4, pp. 399–446.

Mazower, M. (ed.) (1997) *The Policing of Politics in the Twentieth Century*, Providence RI: Berghahn Books.

Parsons, T. (1971) *The System of Modern Societies*, Englewood Cliffs NJ: Prentice-Hall.

Pratt, J. (1999) 'Governmentality, Neo-liberalism and Dangerousness', in R. Smandych (ed.), *Governable Places: Readings on Governmentality and Crime Control*, Aldershot: Ashgate.

Reiner, R. (1988) 'British Criminology and the State', in P. Rock (ed.), *A History of British Criminology*, Oxford: Oxford University Press.

Ruggie, J. G. (1993) 'Territoriality and Beyond: Problematizing Modernity in International Relations', *International Organization*, Vol. 47, No. 1, pp. 139–74.

Shawcross, W. (1979) *Sideshow: Kissinger, Nixon and the Destruction of Cambodia*, London: André Deutsch.

Sheptycki, J. W. E. (1997) 'Insecurity, Risk Suppression and Segregation: Some Reflections on Policing in the Transnational Age', *Theoretical Criminology*, Vol. 1, No. 3, pp. 303–15.

Sheptycki, J. W. E. (1998a) 'Policing, Postmodernism and Transnationalisation', *British Journal of Criminology*, Vol. 38, No. 3, pp. 485–503.

Sheptycki, J. W. E. (1998b) 'Reflections on the Transnationalisation of Policing: The Case of the RCMP and Serial Killers', *International Journal of the Sociology of Law*, Vol. 26, pp. 17–34.

Sheptycki, J. W. E. (2000) 'Editorial Reflections on Intelligence-Led Policing', *A Policing and Society Special Issue, Intelligence-Led Policing*, Vol. 9, No. 4. pp. 311–14.

South, N. (1988) *Policing for Profit: The Private Security Sector*, London: Sage.

Spitzer, S. and Scull, A. (1977) 'Privatisation and Capitalist Development: The Case of Private Police', *Social Problems*, Vol. 25, No. 1, pp. 8–29.

Stenning, P. and Shearing, C. (1980) 'The Quiet Revolution: The Nature, Development and General Legal Implications of Private Policing in Canada', *Criminal Law Quarterly*, Vol. 22, pp. 220–48.

Thurlow, R. (1994) *The Secret State: British Internal Security in the Twentieth Century*, Oxford: Basil Blackwell.

Tilley, C. (1975) *The Formation of States in Western Europe*, Princeton NJ: Princeton University Press.

Tugendhat, C. (1971) *The Multinationals*, London: Eyre and Spottiswoode.

Waltz, K. (1959) *Man, the State and War*, New York: Columbia University Press.

Waltz, K. (1979) *Theory of International Politics*, New York: Random House.

Whitaker, R. and Marcuse, G. (1994) *Cold War Canada: The Making of a National Insecurity State, 1945–1957*, Toronto: University of Toronto Press.

Yoshida, N. (1999) 'Taming the Japanese Security Industry', *Policing and Society*, Vol. 9, No. 3, pp. 241–62.

1 Transnational private policing

The impact of global commercial security

Les Johnston

Introduction

In recent years there has been considerable speculation about the prospects for transnational policing. During the same period there has also been growing interest in the expansion of private policing. Surprisingly, there has been little attempt to consider these issues together, the debate on transnational policing having been largely limited to an analysis of developments within the public police sector. The aim of this chapter is to put right that omission by examining the nature and significance of transnational commercial security.

Before proceeding, it is necessary to discuss some terms ('policing', 'transnational') and provide a rudimentary theoretical context for the discussion which follows. As for the first of these, a few, brief comments will suffice. Policing is concerned with the provision of 'guarantees' or 'assurances' of security (Shearing 1992). As such, it may be undertaken by a wide range of agents including state police, private citizens and commercial companies. One implication of this definition is that policing has to be understood not as the action of a particular body (the state police), but as the interaction of the various bodies which contribute to security. In that respect, policing is a governmental problem – one concerned with the organisation and management of security networks – rather than simply a 'criminological' one.

Transnational policing involves the provision of security across national boundaries. Debate about the transnational character of policing has, so far, focused on developments within and between public police forces. At the formal level, transnational initiatives have been of two types: either policing by national or sub-national bodies, in cooperation with similar bodies, across national boundaries; or policing by genuinely supranational bodies. The former has been more prevalent than the latter, though whether such international (sometimes intergovernmental) initiatives are genuinely transnational remains open to question (Sheptycki 1995). As for the latter, where supranational organisations exist, they have tended to engage in the collection, collation and dissemination of intelligence, rather than in operational policing proper. Sheptycki (1996) reminds us that developments at the informal level are also significant, a point confirmed by the fact that transnational legal practice is shaped, more and more, by transnational police practice. Thus, for example, in the field of drugs enforcement, techniques of 'controlled delivery' (allowing illicit shipments to proceed in order to secure evidence against 'big fish'), though very often not legally prescripted, are, increasingly, sanctioned by prosecutors and members of the judiciary.

While transnational public policing is a relatively new phenomenon, the commercial security market is already dominated by a small number of transnational companies. These multifunctional organisations form complex transnational security networks by virtue of the interaction of their parent companies and branch plants with other commercial and non-commercial security providers. Significantly, their activities – discussed later in the chapter – both transcend and penetrate the state. On the one hand, they perform security functions 'both in between and outside of state spaces' (Kempa et al. 1999: 213). On the other hand, they are called upon by governments to undertake what are, traditionally, considered to be core state functions.

It is important to locate these developments in the theoretical context of late modernity, since this context is discussed in the final section. The formation of state police in the nineteenth century was linked to the establishment of the modern state and to the consolidation of modern society. This modernising project was a product of post-Enlightenment values (regarding rational action, scientific knowledge and behavioural predictability) which defined 'the social' as a discrete field of activity (to be studied by human scientists), and declared 'the state' to be a core apparatus for the governance of social life. Accordingly, the state police's mandate was defined, not just in criminological terms, but also in moral ones – a point exemplified by their role as 'domestic missionaries' (Storch 1976). In effect, uniformed police officers served as the routine embodiment of state sovereignty, personifying public authority at street level by virtue of their possession of constabulary powers.

This state-centred view of the governance of social life remained relatively sacrosanct until undermined by neo-liberalism. Early analysis of the neo-liberal project focused, understandably, on the policy of economic privatisation. Yet, it was clear from the outset that neo-liberalism aspired not only to the 'sale of the family silver', but also to the wholesale 'reinvention of government' (Osborne and Gaebler 1993). Accordingly, the privatisation of policing was more than a series of economic reforms. Rather, it consisted of a complex mixture of commercial, municipal and citizen-based initiatives, occurring at a variety of sectoral and spatial locations, some of which involved the dispersal of responsibility for security to regions outside the confines of the state (Johnston 1992). Neo-liberalism had major implications for both the state and society. On the one hand, demands to 'turn back the clock' and re-impose welfare-liberal modes of governance proved untenable. 'Bringing the state back in' was an impossible solution since the morphology of 'the state' was profoundly affected by the neo-liberal reforms (Johnston 1999). On the other hand if, as was suggested, society was fragmenting into a plurality of diverse communities and interest groups (Rose 1996), the coherence of 'the social' as an organising principle for governing human relations was also cast into doubt. Together, the implication of these developments was clear. The fundamental assumption of modern governance – that the state was the essential apparatus for governing social life – was doubly unsustainable.

Analysing transnational private policing in the light of this debate raises certain issues. For example, there has been much speculation about the changing 'sectoral' balance arising from the growth of private (commercial) as opposed to public (state) police (Shearing and Stenning 1987; South 1988; Johnston 1992). One of the problems with this 'sectoral' mode of analysis, however, is the adequacy of the public–private distinction itself. For one thing, debates about late modernity call into question the view that the state remains the embodiment of public/collective life when human relations are, increasingly, contained within a discourse of 'consumerism' and located in the market-place. In this regard, some writers have pointed to the growth of 'corporate governments' (Shearing 1992), raising the question of whether they possess the potential to become genuine 'corporate communities' with 'corporate citizens' (Elkins 1995). Behind this is a question about whether, under the right governmental conditions, commercial interests can be marshalled so as to contribute to the collective good. The issue of whether the growth of transnational commercial security can – notwithstanding its dangers – have positive potential is considered later.

The following discussion is divided into four sections. The first provides some basic information on the size and structure of the commercial security market. Section Two considers some leading transnational contract security companies. Section Three analyses the activities undertaken by these companies, paying particular attention to those which signify the emergence of corporate forms of governance in areas where states lack exclusive sovereignty. The final section explores the theoretical implications of these developments and assesses some of the problems and prospects posed by the expansion of transnational commercial security.

The commercial security market

Though organisations such as Pinkerton, Wells Fargo and Securicor had their origins in the nineteenth century and in the early years of the twentieth, it is during the last three decades that commercial security has enjoyed its most sustained growth. Cunningham et al. (1990) estimated that gross revenue from sales and services in the US contract sector amounted to $37.9 billion in 1990 with annual growth rates running at 10 per cent. Latest projections suggest that overall growth will continue at around 8.5 per cent per annum until 2002 with average annual revenue amounting to almost twice that generated by taxes for public law enforcement (Kempa et al. 1999).

The market in Europe is by no means as large as that in the USA, but it is undergoing rapid expansion. Research undertaken by McAlpine, Thorpe and Warrier (MTW) (Narayan 1994a) estimated that the total market for security products and services in France, Germany, Italy, Spain and the UK stood at £11.2 billion in 1992. MTW predicted that the market would grow at an average rate of 6 per cent per annum, reaching a total of £14 billion by 1996. Security services – primarily manned guarding and cash-in-transit – retained the largest proportion of the overall market (£4.3 billion) while electronic systems held a market share of £3.9 billion and physical products took up the remaining £3 billion. Particularly high annual growth rates were found for CCTV (11.4 per cent), integrated systems (11.8 per cent) and access control (7.7 per cent).

The ability of multinational companies to penetrate domestic security markets is noted in a recent report on the European access control sector. Here, particular reference is made to the growing influence of multinational companies such as Group 4, Chubb, Abloy, Hengsler and Siemens (Frost and Sullivan 1995). Such penetration is not, however, restricted to Europe. Cunningham et al. (1990) note that between 1985 and 1989 British, Swiss, Australian, and Japanese corporations invested over $4 billion in American security companies. Indeed, almost a quarter of sales and acquisitions occurring in the USA during this period involved foreign investment, the dominant source being the UK.

While the countries of North Central and North-west Europe have experienced significant levels of overall growth, those of Eastern and Southern Europe and Asia – where the industry is more recently established – have seen greater degrees of relative growth (Kempa et al. 1999). Though the first Japanese commercial security company was only established in 1962, by 1993 more than 7,000 security companies employed more than 320,000 guards, a figure exceeding the combined authorised strength of the National and Prefectural Police by over 60,000 (Miyazawa 1991; National Police Agency 1994). Since the passing of legislation in 1981, rapid development has also taken place in Turkey where, by 1993, 2,227 companies employed almost 35,000 people (Kempa et al. 1999). In India it is estimated that contract security personnel now outnumber public police by a factor of 2:1 (ibid.).

Local, regional and transnational security companies are also active in many African countries including Zimbabwe, Nigeria and Kenya. However, by far the most dramatic growth has occurred in post-apartheid South Africa where the industry now has an estimated value of almost Rand 6 billion. Here, official figures show that with 4,345 companies employing 363,928 registered guards, numbers employed in commercial security exceed members of the South African Police Service by a ratio of about 3:1 (de Waard 1999). Following escalating levels of crime, South Africa has been a particularly fertile market for overseas security companies, many of them British. In the mid-1990s the (Conservative) UK government appointed a full-time export promoter to encourage investment in the South African crime prevention market and Britain became a leading supplier of electronic security products, such as surveillance cameras, alarms and infra-red detectors. Subsequently, companies like Chubb became involved in the provision of armed defence systems, supplying SWAT-like 'reaction teams'– armed with automatic weapons – to victimised customers. Commenting on these developments, a representative of Chubb noted that 'British companies see South Africa as a growing market, whereas the British one may be saturated' (cited in Woolf 1996: 1).

Transnational contract security companies

Transnational contract security companies have certain common features. They generate high revenues, high rates of annual growth and high profits. They engage in dynamic market activity through acquisitions, sales and joint ventures. They seek to penetrate new markets, an increasing number of which are overseas. They are, more often than not, multifunctional organisations engaged in the provision of a variety of services. Group 4 Securitas (International) operates in over 30 countries, employs more than 50,000 people and has an annual turnover exceeding £600 million. Some of its UK subsidiaries include Group 4 (International) Corrections, Group 4 Remand Services, Group 4 Store Detectives, Guardforce International, Secom Security and Securitas Technology (Kompass 1994). In the last decade the group has entered the growing Eastern European market. In the Czech Republic, a workforce of over 3,000 is engaged in the provision of physical security, cash transportation and the installation and maintenance of technical security systems. Among the company's major clients are energy companies, nuclear power stations and chemical plants.

The Securicor Group plc (whose web page is headed by the message 'Global Expertise, Local Understanding') is a holding company whose subsidiaries provide a wide variety of services: express parcel delivery, cash transportation and processing, mobile and static guarding, secure IT services, vehicle fleet servicing, mobile communications, telecommunication products, electronic surveillance and alarms, stolen vehicle recovery, the financing, construction and design of prisons, immigration services, prisoner transfer, electronic monitoring, hotels and leisure facilities, office cleaning and recruitment services. In 1992 the group employed almost 41,000 staff and had sales of £583 million. By 1997 sales had risen to £1,350 million (Extel 1993; Key British Enterprises 1994; UK Business Park: 1998).

The extent of Securicor's overseas activity is striking, the bulk of which has occurred in South Africa (*Security Gazette*, Summer 1995: 89), South-east Asia and the Americas. In 1990 Securicor established a joint venture with Jardine Pacific to form the largest security services company in South-east Asia. It now employs 8,000 people in Hong Kong, Malaysia and Macau. Subsequently, joint ventures have been set up in Indonesia (*Professional Security*, November 1992: 31) and in Thailand. The latter company, with 6,000 staff, is the country's largest security business (*International Security Review*, Autumn 1993: 12). Another agreement with Jardine Pacific led to the formation of Securicor Taiwan Ltd (*Security Gazette*, August 1994: 11). Joint ventures have also been set up in the Caribbean where, in 1994, an office was opened in Georgetown, Guyana, to provide monitoring, cash-in-transit and guarding (*Security Gazette*, November 1994: 11). A similar venture has been established in Costa Rica as part of Securicor's programme to establish bases in Central American and Caribbean countries which have stable security markets and are linked to the US dollar (*Security Gazette*, February 1995: 11).

North American-based companies display similar expansionist tendencies. In 1997 the US security company ADT merged with Tyco International Ltd, adopting the latter's name. Tyco is a diversified manufacturing and service company specialising in disposable medical supplies, flow control products, electrical components and fire and security services (Tyco International Ltd 1998). The Fire and Security Services Group markets electronic security products world-wide under a number of well-known brand names including ADT, Modern, Sonitrol and Thorn Security. In 1998 the Group acquired Holmes Protection and Wells Fargo Alarm, two US security monitoring companies; CIPE, a French company, thereby making Tyco the number one security monitoring company in Europe; and a number of small security companies in Australia, New Zealand, Singapore and Argentina. In 1998 the Fire and Security Services Group reported earnings of $654.9 million, a 45 per cent increase on the previous year. During the same period sales grew by 14 per cent to $4.74 billion (Tyco International Ltd 1999). It is anticipated that 1999 revenues will exceed $17 billion (*Boston Globe* 1998).

Tyco's Chairman, L. Dennis Kozlowski, anticipates that 'as security concerns rise and demographics change around the globe', these high levels of growth will continue. This is particularly true of the global home security market, Tyco's field of specialism, where there has been little market penetration: only 20 per cent coverage in the USA, less than 5 per cent in Europe; and under 2 per cent in Latin America – an area particularly ripe for expansion. Some of that market penetration will depend upon the development of new technologies for newly defined security problems. For example, Kozlowski notes the company's recent success in marketing sophisticated motion-detectors for use in the domestic environment: 'parents can now be notified every time a child arrives home safely' (Tyco International Ltd 1998: 17–18).

The Wackenhut Corporation was founded in 1954 and now employs 56,000 staff in nearly 50 countries on six continents. In 1961 company revenue amounted to $5.4 million, all of it from North American Operations. By 1976 revenue had risen to $123 million, 90 per cent of it from North American Operations, the remainder from Wackenhut International. By 1995 North American Operations accounted for 74 per cent of the Corporation's total revenue of $797 million, the remainder coming from Wackenhut International (14 per cent) and Wackenhut Corrections (12 per cent). The Corporation is now divided into four major operational units, each with functional subdivisions. North

American Operations consists of a Security Services Division (providing physical security and investigative services), Wackenhut Services Inc. (providing protective services, court security, emergency medical services and rescue services to government agencies), a Nuclear Services Division (protecting nuclear power plants from disruptive threats and theft of nuclear material), Correctional Foodservice Management and the Wackenhut Training Institute. Wackenhut International consists of an International Trading Corporation (providing clients with state-of-the-art security products) and an International Division which provides a full range of security services to clients in almost fifty countries. Wackenhut Correction consists of a Correctional Division, offering a full range of services for the financing, design, construction and management of prisons; a Development Unit which serves as a general contractor in developing new facilities; and a healthcare division (Atlantic Shores Healthcare) which provides comprehensive mental healthcare services to prison facilities. Wackenhut Resources provides a full range of human resources, employee leasing and staffing services to business (Wackenhut 1998).

In 1997 Wackenhut revenues passed $1 billion, a 24 per cent increase on the previous fiscal year. During the year the company's North American Operations grew by 8 per cent, its International Operations by 13 per cent and its revenue from Corrections by 50 per cent. Wackenhut International recently secured contracts with the Buenos Aires subway transit system; the Puerto Rico Telephone Company; the Puerto Rico Building Authority; three Guatemalan banks; steel mills in Venezuela; General Motors facilities in Peru, Venezuela and Ecuador and an electrical corporation in Morocco. Cash-in-transit operations expanded into Guatemala and the Dominican Republic (Wackenhut 1998).

One of Wackenhut's main North American rivals, the Pinkerton Corporation, founded in 1850, now employs 47,000 people in more than 250 offices in the USA, Canada, Latin America, Europe and Asia. The company had revenues in excess of $1 billion during the fiscal year ending 1997, an increase of 11 per cent on the previous year's figures. Clients include General Motors, AT&T, IBM, Hewlett Packard and Proctor & Gamble and, overall, it is claimed that Pinkerton represents 82 per cent of the US *Fortune 1,000* companies. The company claims to have 'an aggressive acquisition program focusing on high margin security businesses, as well as growth by foreign expansion' (Pinkerton 1998).

This last comment should be remembered in considering a final company, Securitas, founded in Helsingborg in 1934. Though, for many years, Securitas restricted its operations to Sweden, a massive programme of expansion took place in the last decade of the twentieth century with acquisitions in Norway, Denmark and Portugal and a new operation being established in Hungary (all during 1989); further acquisitions were made in France, Switzerland, Spain, Austria and Germany (1992), Finland (1993), Britain, Poland and Estonia (1996), and Sweden and France (1997). Recently, two major European rivals, Proteg and Raab Karcher Sicherheit, were also acquired. Following the purchase of these two companies, Securitas claims to account for 10 per cent of total sales by European security companies (Securitas 1998). Annual profits rose by 17 per cent during 1996, advancing from SKr 472 million to SKr 550 million ($74.1 million) (McIvor 1997). Commenting on these figures, the company's Chief Executive, Thomas Berglund, stated that the European market was growing by between 5 per cent and 10 per cent per annum and predicted that its current value (SKr 164 billion) would double within a decade: 'The size of the market is no restriction . . . the amount we can grow . . . is more a question of our own energies' (cited in McIvor 1997).

This comment proved an apposite one. In February 1999 – as this chapter was being completed – Securitas paid SKr 3 billion (£230 million) for the acquisition of Pinkerton. The purchase produces the world's largest security company with combined sales of SKr 27 billion and 114,000 employees. By combining the core activities of Securitas (alarms, cash-in-transit, guarding) with those of Pinkerton (pre-employment screening, risk assessment, integrated security systems) it also produces a company with massive 'global reach'. Commenting on the acquisition, James McCloskey, Chief Financial Officer of Pinkerton – whose brand name is retained in the restructured company – noted that the purchase would bring Securitas 'an incredible array of global customers' (cited in Burt 1999).

Transnational security activities

Sheptycki (1995) lists a number of problems which are linked to the growth of transnational public policing. These include international terrorism and espionage, drugs trafficking, arms trafficking, corporate crime, environmental crime and transnational fraud. Most of these areas may also be regarded as growth markets for commercial security. Consider drugs and terrorism. Cunningham et al. (1990) estimated that the drug-testing market, alone, could be worth $1billion by the year 2000. Other revenue sources will include the increased use of undercover agents in drugs intelligence and surveillance work, the provision of drug prevention and treatment programmes and the manufacture and sale of drug detection equipment. They also note that increased revenues for security companies might arise from various anti-terrorist initiatives including the provision of security systems at airports, risk analysis and crisis management services, executive protection programmes, the manufacture, sale and monitoring of specialised technical equipment and facility hardening.

Other opportunities are also emerging. Global population movement – through travel, tourism and migration – is already being regulated more by commercial than by state police. Airline security, in particular, has become a virtual private monopoly. As Kirby (1993) points out, in the late 1980s a number of private aviation security companies were established in response to an immediate need for the major international carriers to counter the threat of terrorist bombings and hijackings. Had that private sector response not been forthcoming, 'many international routes [would have been] under the threat of closure' (p. 22). In addition to dealing with airborne terrorism, private security companies have also inherited the task of policing migrants and refugees. Here, in particular, governments 'have passed the responsibility for preventing the transportation of passengers with improper documentation to the air carriers' (ibid.). Developments like these are indicative of an emergent 'corporate governance' residing at the interstices of the state and the market. This can be illustrated by considering three further examples.

Business risks

Anticipating business risks and minimising the losses arising from them is the essence of commercial security practice. The opening up of Eastern Europe during the 1990s spawned a number of security companies specialising in the anticipation, assessment and minimisation of the personal and corporate risks associated with entering new foreign markets. One such company, Control Risks Group Ltd, describes itself as an 'international political and security risk consultancy' offering a range of services for those contemplating investing in Russia and the former Soviet republics. Those services include vetting the personal and professional backgrounds of key local individuals; vetting the market reputations and business histories of potential corporate partners; assessing the local political scene; giving information on safe local hotels and unsafe city areas; and advising in hostage negotiation should it be required (Rainey 1996). Pinkerton offers similar services on a world-wide basis. Pinkerton International (Asia), for instance, provides security surveys, personnel screening, executive protection, 'due diligence' checks on potential partners, forensic audits, crisis management and contingency planning facilities, investigative services, armed guards and a variety of other services to multinational companies investing in the People's Republic of China, Indonesia, Korea, Malaysia, the Philippines, Singapore, Taiwan and Thailand (Pinkerton 1998).

One critical factor in these developments has been the commodification of information. Manning notes that the US government, in co-operation with large corporations (many of them part of the defence industry) 'has broadened its definition of the national interest to include "information" (read: industrial secrets and ideas with "R and D" potential)' (Manning 1996: 4, and see Manning, this volume). In effect, Manning suggests, governments now include proprietary corporate information within the scope of 'the national interest' and actively seek to ensure its effective policing. This task of information policing is, of course, undertaken by corporate bodies, Pinkerton again providing the model through its Washington based Global Intelligence Services group (GIS).

GIS functions to inform business executives about any international threats which might affect their interests or compromise the safety of their personnel. GIS staff are specialists in information analysis, criminal investigation, counter-intelligence, anti-terrorism, counter-espionage and threat analysis. The great majority have previously occupied senior positions in the military – particularly in the US Air Force Office of Special Investigations (AFOSI). The Managing Director of GIS directed the AFOSI anti-terrorism programme for four years and also commanded its Iran unit for a similar period. The Chief Consultant retired as a Colonel in the US Air Force, having served as both US Advisor to the Vietnamese Air Force Security Office (with a counter-intelligence brief) and as a Special Agent with AFOSI. Two Senior Consultants have previous experience with AFOSI, one as Director for Research, the other as a counter-intelligence liaison officer in Grenada. Another served as Director for Counter-intelligence in the Office of the Secretary of State for Defense (Pinkerton 1998). It should not be assumed, however, that these interstitial links between commercial security, government and the military are peculiar to Pinkerton. Wackenhut's Board of Directors includes a former special agent of the FBI (Chairman George R. Wackenhut, himself), a retired lieutenant-general from the US Army, a retired Marine Corps four star general, a former Under Secretary of the US Air Force and a past Governor of South Carolina (Wackenhut 1998).

Custodial and correctional facilities

Commercial involvement in the control of so-called 'problem' populations is by no means new, the UK's Immigration Detention Centres having been run by Securicor and Group 4 since 1970. The invisibility of immigrants and asylum-seekers from public gaze was probably a factor which appealed to commercial security companies looking for a 'foot in the door' of the corrections market. Green (1989) suggests that Group 4 undercut Securicor in 1989 – and, in so doing, took on an unprofitable contract – in order to establish its credentials with the Home Office, in anticipation of the future private prisons programme. This was an astute move since the privatisation of corrections moved on at a rapid pace, both in Britain and elsewhere.

In Britain, the old penal lobby of criminal justice professionals, voluntary and statutory agencies quickly gave way to a new policy-making elite composed of representatives from the building industry, banks and commercial security companies (Johnston 1992). In 1992 a new remand prison (the Wolds) was opened under Group 4 management. In the following five years a further ten institutions were either opened, planned or under development. As Morgan (1997) points out, after some early difficulties, these facilities appear to be setting some high standards, though concern remains about whether the commercial sector may cream off selected institutions, leaving the state to manage more costly facilities. That possibility aside, it is interesting to note that the UK Home Secretary, Jack Straw, began his term of office expressing a moral repugnance for prison privatisation and, under continuing pressure to find accommodation, not least for illegal immigrants awaiting extradition, gradually shifted towards a commitment to further expansion under precisely this rubric.

These developments are by no means peculiar to Britain, similar ones having occurred in the USA, Australia and New Zealand. Harding (1997) suggests that, within three years, 20 per cent of Australian prisoners could be held in private facilities, the highest proportion for any country. Though, in the USA, percentage proportions are much lower than this, the massive – and expanding – prison population offers huge financial potential for the commercial security sector. As a senior executive of the Corrections Corporation of America, the leading North American consortium, stated, 'There are powerful market forces driving our industry, and its potential has barely been touched' (cited in Harding 1997: 4). In fact, that potential has already begun to be realised by companies like Wackenhut. Wackenhut Corrections was established in 1984, its first custodial contracts – as with Group 4 and

Securicor in the UK – being with the Immigration and Naturalization Service. By 1995 the Corrections Division accounted for 12 per cent of Wackenhut's $797 million revenue. In 1997 the annual revenue for corrections rose by 50 per cent (following a 38 per cent increase the previous year) to account for 19 per cent of a total company revenue of $1,127 million. To put those figures in perspective, revenue from this *single* source had now almost doubled the revenue from *all* company sources recorded in 1976 (Wackenhut 1998).

Added to that, there is the potential for new markets. By the late 1990s Wackenhut Corrections already had more than 30,000 'beds' under contract in forty-six facilities in the USA, Puerto Rico, England, Scotland and Australia. In 1997 the South African government released tender documents inviting the major security companies to bid for the financing, construction and management of seven prisons at an estimated cost of £208 million. Once undertaken, these contracts would put South Africa amongst the world leaders in prison privatisation, initially providing 10,000 new prison places. However, the government's long-term objective has been to provide for a further 50,000 private places, enabling it to withdraw completely from financing further construction (Matthews 1997).

National security policy

If further proof is needed of the emergence of corporate governance, one only has to look at national security policy – arguably the most basic of all state functions – whose commercial penetration is well under way. This is particularly apparent in regions where the police and the military are ineffective or where long-standing political or military disputes remain unresolved. Recall when, in Papua New Guinea, the army rebelled against politicians who employed Sandline International, a British company, to put down a long-running rebellion on the island of Bougainville. Sandline's Chief Executive, Lieutenant-Colonel Tim Spicer, was arrested and put on trial, while the Papuan Prime Minister, Sir Julius Chan, was forced to resign. Bougainville is a province rich in minerals and it is alleged that one of Sandline's objectives was to wrest control of the world's biggest copper mine from the dissidents, enabling the Port Moresby government to give a significant interest in the mine to the company controlling Sandline (Findlay 1999). However, it should not be assumed that these adventures are merely the product of corporate ambition. When Sandline admitted to supplying weapons in order to help restore the

Kabbah regime in Sierra Leone, it claimed that senior British diplomats, seeking to bolster Britain's commercial interests, were also privy to the action (Russell 1998).

Whether this allegation is true or not there is undeniable complicity between the government and similar 'professional services companies' in the US. The best known of these is Military Professional Resources Inc. (MPRI), a company engaged primarily in military-related contracting in the US and international defence markets. The company was established in 1987 by eight former senior military officers and its core business includes 'training, equipping, force design and management, professional development, concepts and doctrine, organisational and operational assistance, quick reaction military contractual support, and democracy transition assistance programmes for the military forces of emerging republics' (MPRI 1998). In 1997, the company had over 400 employees and its volume of business exceeded $48 million. In late 1995 MPRI undertook its first major foreign training operation, helping to 'turn the Croatian army from a rag-bag militia into a formidable fighting force' (Alexander 1997). In the course of fulfilling this contract, however, French and British officials accused MPRI of helping to plan the Croatian invasion of Bosnia, a charge denied by the company (US News and World Report 1997).

The closeness of ties between the Pentagon and MPRI are no better illustrated than in its involvement in Bosnia and Angola. In Bosnia the Clinton Administration urged the Federation to enlist the services of a private company in order to equalise the conflict between it and the Bosnian Serbs. Under the terms of the contract, valued at 'tens of millions of dollars', the company sent more than 170 former military trainers to restructure the Bosnian Army. Finance for the project was obtained from a number of Islamic countries while, at the same time, the Bosnian Army received more than $100 million worth of surplus military equipment from the US government (US News and World Report 1997). US officials stated that the intervention programme was effective in supporting two objectives of US regional policy. First, it put pressure on Muslim and Croat forces to begin merging into a single army. Secondly, the promise of US military assistance pressured the Sarajevo authorities to break off channels of Iranian arms and training opened during the war. A joke made in Bosnia, at the time, was that MPRI really stood for 'Military Professionals Replacing Iran' (Graham 1997).

The work of private military contractors has caused some concern in government circles, one anonymous official declaring

I have a problem with the privatization of US foreign policy and national security policy . . . It gives you what the intelligence community have had for a long period of time: plausible deniability. It is a way of getting things done that the administration doesn't have to go to the Hill or to the American public to talk about.

(*US News and World Report* 1997)

Despite these reservations, however, the US government played a direct role in lobbying the Angolan government on behalf of MPRI, the Angolans having originally hired a South African company, Executive Outcomes (EO), to reverse the military gains of the UNITA army. US government pressure eventually forced the Angolan and South African Governments to replace EO with MPRI.

Executive Outcomes was established in 1989 as a wholly owned South African company, drawing many of its personnel from the police and defence forces after their 'down-sizing'. Subsequently, it has operated in support of armed forces, private corporations and law enforcement agencies in Southern Africa, West Africa, the Far East and South America. EO's first contracts were to develop special warfare packages on covert operations for the South African Defence Force. Later, work was undertaken for the mining industry (countering white-collar crime and trafficking of high-value commodities) and for a South American drugs enforcement agency ('discretionary warfare' against growers). EO publicity material comments on the worldwide tendency towards the privatisation of security and predicts that 'future peacekeeping/refugee operations will be conducted more and more by companies like EO' (Executive Outcomes 1998).

Richard Cornwell of the African Institute in Pretoria has suggested that these developments indicate the privatisation of war and security, 'companies [taking] their own private armies with them to places where state control is non-existent' (cited in Alexander 1997). There is much truth in this statement. However, it is necessary to add two caveats. First, unlike mercenaries of the past, the personnel employed by these companies have impeccable military credentials (Keegan 1998). Secondly, because of this, they enjoy the endorsement of government, being integrated with all aspects of security policy – from the furtherance of foreign policy objectives by alternative means, to the exercise of informal justice in the world of global crime. In effect, these companies 'reach the parts that other agencies cannot reach', though often with the complicity of government.

Conclusion

Two interrelated issues arise in respect of transnational commercial security. How should it be theorised? And how should it be evaluated? As to the first of these, what little theoretical analysis there has been, refers mainly to the privatisation of corrections. Baldry, commenting on the Australian experience, contends that prison privatisation is simply the most recent attempt by US transnational corporations to 'create markets for their products where they are non-existent' (Baldry 1996: 161). The result is that Australia's relationship to the USA is, increasingly, one of a client state contained within a neo-colonialist framework: 'Australian states find themselves . . . caught up in the international corrections complex . . . this is comparable with the neo-colonialist nature of the US nuclear power industry, chemical and medical corporations' (p. 172).

Lilley and Knepper (1992) argue that the international corrections market is dominated by the US 'corrections-commercial complex', an alliance of commercial, governmental and professional agencies, enjoying close links with the international military–industrial complex. Such is the power of this alliance that it is able to function as a 'sub-government', effectively determining key elements of US and UK corrections policy. A further critical issue is transnational ownership. During the late 1980s the Corrections Corporation of America received British investment through Enskilda Industries, the London merchant bankers, while other British companies bought directly into the US security market. Similar patterns of transnational investment occurred with electronic monitoring, British, American and Japanese electronic multinationals combining to create new markets in Europe and Asia. The electronics market, in particular, proved a fruitful source of investment for defence contractors, such as Racal-Chubb and GEC Plessey, in their search to benefit from the 'peace dividend': 'security firms . . . which specialise in technology for "access control", "alarm sensors", "closed circuit TV", "manned security" . . . and . . . "perimeter protection" just as eagerly sell these products to the military as they do to prison warders and shopping malls' (p. 184).

Though these analyses are similar in many respects, they differ slightly in how they assess the impact of transnational developments on governance. Baldry's (1996) unequivocal view is that the power of US capital eradicates the sovereignty of nation-states, reducing them to mere clients. The effect is to replace national state sovereignty with the sovereignty of transnational capital. Lilley and Knepper's (1992) position is rather more guarded. Their claim, that transnational corporations function as *sub*-governments, suggests a more variegated and diverse governmental model in which policy is the product of interaction between a plurality of state, commercial, military and professional bodies. In effect, this position opens the door to diversity, then closes it rapidly, postulating that diverse interests coalesce into a unified power bloc. However, such a position is difficult to maintain under contemporary conditions and raises questions about how we are to understand late modernity.

The modern nation-state was marked by the development of two institutional complexes: military organisations, whose task was to secure the state's territorial integrity; and police organisations, whose task was to maintain internal security (Dandeker 1990). State monopoly of national and sub-national security (through the state police) has now been undermined by the growth of diverse modes of commercial and voluntary provision (Johnston 1992). Similar diversity is emerging at the transnational level, one aspect of which – commercialisation – has been discussed in this chapter. These developments should come as no surprise since diversity is one of the key correlates of globalisation. Globalisation, in turn, is a core constituent of late modernity and a critical factor in transnational development. Far from producing uniformity (transnational capital neither eradicates nation-states nor produces a transnational 'superstate'), globalisation combines opposing trends: organisational centralisation and decentralisation; structural fragmentation and consolidation; cultural homogeneity and heterogeneity. In short, globalisation builds diversity into governance. As Nederveen Pierterse (1995) argues, it involves the emergence of new organisational complexes at transnational, international, national, regional, municipal and local levels. Such complexes are, in turn, intersected by functional networks of business corporations, international agencies, professional organisations and others to produce 'two interactive worlds with overlapping memberships: a state-centric world, in which the primary actors are national, and a multi-centric world of diverse actors such as corporations, international organisations, ethnic groups, churches' (p. 50).

Diversification of government was, of course, one of the objectives of the neo-liberal project. Yet, this process of governmental 're-invention' (Osborne and Gaebler 1993) entailed only a circumscribed diversity. Government was to be dispersed, but within clearly defined limits so that the state would retain control of 'steering', leaving others to do the 'rowing' ('rule at a distance'). In retrospect, it is clear that this approach overestimated the state's directive capacity. From what has been seen in this chapter, it is clear that, in the security field, diversity has already exceeded the boundaries of the neo-liberal project: 'non-state entities are not simply mobilized by the state, but have themselves developed the capacity to mobilize and direct other resources' (Shearing and Wood forthcoming). What diversity implies, then, is neither 'state rule at a distance', nor the subjugation of the state to transnational capital, nor, indeed, the domination of a unified power elite, but a changing morphology of governance in which partly fragmented states interact with commercial, civil and voluntary bodies both within and across national jurisdictional boundaries.

Taking this governmental complex into account, how then should the growth of transnational commercial security be evaluated? It is tempting to regard the developments described in this chapter as mere confirmation of an unbridled and unaccountable corporate power riding roughshod over national and local interests. Further fuel may be added to this view by allegations of corporate impropriety. Wackenhut has, for example, been at the centre of two such charges. In one, a US newspaper alleged that the company was profiting from programmes which were supposed to be break-even operations, that it had diverted $700,000 from drug programmes at a Texas treatment centre, and that auditors had identified $307,000 in questionable overhead costs (Dimmock 1995). A second allegation related to the company's contract with the Alyeska Pipeline Service Company, a consortium involved in Alaskan oil exploration and extraction. In 1991 the House Interior Committee met to hear allegations about covert surveillance said to have been conducted by Wackenhut against Charles Hamel, an environmental 'whistle-blower'. Several ex-Wackenhut employees testified to having been involved in dubious activities aimed to discredit Hamel and Alyeska employees who had accused the company of environmentally unsound practices. Wackenhut had also, apparently, used unlicensed investigators in undertaking this work (US House of Representatives 1991).

Neither specific allegations of impropriety, nor general concerns about corporate hegemony should be taken lightly. Yet, these concerns have to be balanced with other considerations. For one thing, it is a mistake to regard globalisation – of which transnationalisation is a part – as a homogeneous force certain to eradicate local autonomy. Robertson (1995) is typical of many writers on global themes who insist that globalisation – or 'glocalisation' as he would prefer it – also involves the invention and reinvention of the local. For, just as global forces impact on the local, so local actions may impact, reciprocally, on the global. ('Think globally, act locally.') Added to that, there is the sheer uncertainty of global futures. It is quite legitimate to express concern about military penetration of civil security (Johnston 1999). Yet, the product of military decision-making is difficult to predict. Radical critics of the 1960s might have seen the US Department of Defense's decision to set up a communication system capable of surviving thermonuclear attack as a manifestation of 'Big Brother'. Today, the internet – while, undoubtedly, a significant source of corporate profit – is regarded as an exemplary form of free expression under late modern conditions.

Finally, any evaluation of transnational commercial security must be prepared to consider its positive potential as well as its obvious resident dangers. In considering such potential, two things are worthy of thought. First, there is no reason, in principle, why commercial security – whether considered at sub-national, national or transnational levels – should be unable to contribute to collective well-being, *provided that it is located within an appropriate governmental regime*. It is, surely, incumbent upon us – given the increasing weakness of the state-society model of governance – to give this matter serious thought. One effect of late modern change is to uncouple the realm of collective action from the public sphere and it is this which provides the rationale behind Elkins's (1995) problematic: can corporate governments become corporate communities with corporate citizens? The mere fact that commercial provision, as presently constituted, may add to the inequitable distribution of security, does not justify dismissal of that question. Rather, the aim should be to consider how an understanding of corporate modes of governance might inform new democratic thinking. Secondly, it is worth considering the 'mentality' of commercial security, something which has not been considered here. The practice of commercial security is informed by a risk-based mentality whose focus is instrumental, calculative, preventative, anticipatory and future-oriented. This risk-based philosophy has already penetrated domestic and transnational policing to a significant degree and critics, rightly, draw attention to the dangers of mere 'actuarial justice' (Hudson 1996). However, there are also benefits attached to risk-based thinking. In particular, risk-reduction is consistent with a penal philosophy less preoccupied with inflicting punishment than with minimising harm. This suggests that, in the future, commercial security may provide new insights for criminology, as well as for democratic theory and practice.

References

Alexander, P. (1997) 'South Africa's Veterans Recruit Army of Outlaws', *Daily Telegraph*, 6 April.

40   *Les Johnston*

Baldry, E. (1996) 'Prison Privateers: Neo-Colonialists in NSW', *Howard Journal*, Vol. 35, No. 2, pp. 161–74.

Boston Globe (1998) 'Tyco International Pays $237m for Entergy Unit', 16 December.

Bowman, E. J. (1996) 'Security Tools up for the Future', *Security Management*, January, pp. 30–4.

Burt, T. (1999) 'Securitas Pays £230m for US Rival Pinkerton', *Financial Times*, 23 February.

Cunningham, W. C., Strauchs, J. J. and Van Meter, C. W. (1990) *Private Security Trends 1970–2000*, Boston: Butterworth-Heinemann.

Dandeker, C. (1990) *Surveillance, Power and Modernity*, Cambridge: Polity Press.

Dimmock, G. (1995) 'Wackenhut Probed for Missing Funds', *Telegraph Journal*, 31 August.

Elkins, D. J. (1995) *Beyond Sovereignty: Territory and Political Economy in the Twenty-first Century*, Toronto: University of Toronto Press.

Executive Outcomes (1998) http://www.eo.com/about/html

Extel (1993) *Extel Financial European Handbook*, Vol. 2, London, June.

Findlay, M. (1999) *The Globalisation of Crime*, Cambridge: Cambridge University Press.

Frost and Sullivan (1995) 'Access Control: a European Market Overview', *International Security Review*, Winter, pp. 17–18.

Graham, B. (1997) 'Ex-GIs Work to Give Bosnian Force a Fighting Chance', *Washington Post*, 29 January.

Green, P. (1989) *Private Sector Involvement in the Immigration Detention Centres*, London: The Howard League for Penal Reform.

Harding, R. W. (1997) *Private Prisons and Public Accountability*, Buckingham: Open University Press.

Hudson, B. (1996) *Understanding Justice*, Buckingham: Open University Press.

Johnston, L. (1992) *The Rebirth of Private Policing*, London: Routledge.

Johnston, L. (1999) *Policing Britain: Risk, Security and Governance*, London: Longman.

Keegan, J. (1998) 'Private Armies Are a Far Cry from the Sixties Dogs of War', *Electronic Telegraph*, Issue 1083, http://www.telegraph.co.uk

Kempa, M., Carrier, R., Wood, J. and Shearing, C. (1999) 'Reflections on the Evolving Concept of "Private Policing"', *European Journal on Criminal Policy and Research*, Vol. 7, No. 1, pp. 197–223.

Key British Enterprises (1994) *Key British Enterprises*, High Wycombe: Dunn and Bradstreet.

Kirby, G. (1993) 'Only One Chance', *Professional Security*, Vol. 3, No. 6, pp. 22–4.

Kompass (1994) (in association with the Confederation of British Industry) *The Authority of British Industry*, East Grinstead: Reed Information Services.

Lilley, J. R. and Knepper, P. (1992) 'An International Perspective on the Privatisation of Corrections', *Howard Journal*, Vol. 31, No. 3, pp. 174–91.

McIvor, G. (1997) 'Acquisitions Drive Growth at Securitas', *Financial Times*, 10 February.

Manning, P. (1996) ' "Global" Transnational Policing: Notes on Changes in the Nature of Social Organization Bearing on Policing', paper presented to the Law and Society Association and Research Committee on the Sociology of Law of the International Sociological Association Joint Meeting, 'Globalisation and the Quest for Justice', Glasgow, Scotland, 10–13 July.

Matthews, R. (1997) 'South Africa Turns to Private Sector for Jails', *Financial Times*, 12 May.

Miyazawa, S. (1991) 'The Private Sector and Law Enforcement in Japan', in W. T. Gormley (ed.), *Privatization and Its Alternative*, Madison: University of Wisconsin Press, pp. 241–57.

Morgan, R. (1997) 'Imprisonment: Current Concerns and a Brief History since 1945', in M. Maguire, R. Morgan and R. Reiner (eds), *The Oxford Handbook of Criminology*, Oxford: Clarendon Press.

MPRI (1998) MPRI Company Info. http://www.mpri.co

Narayan, S. (1994a) 'The West European Market for Security Products and Services', *International Security Review*, Spring, pp. 43–4.

Narayan, S. (1994b) 'An Eye on the Market', *International Security Review*, Winter, pp. 28–9.

National Police Agency (1994) *White Paper on Police 1994 (Excerpt)*, Tokyo: National Police Agency, Government of Japan.

Nederveen Pierterse, J. (1995) 'Global System, Globalization and the Parameters of Modernity', pp. 45–68 in M. Featherstone, S. Lash and R. Robertson (eds) *Global Modernities*, London: Sage.

Osborne, D. and Gaebler, T. (1993) *Reinventing Government*, New York: Plume.

Pinkerton (1998) http://www.pinkerton.co

Rainey, S. (1996) 'Dangerous Liaisons?', *Security Gazette*, April, pp. 12–14.

Robertson, R. (1995) 'Glocalisation: Time–Space and Homogeneity–Heterogeneity', pp. 25–44 in M. Featherstone, S. Lash and R. Robertson (eds), *Global Modernities*, London: Sage.

Rose, N. (1996) 'The Death of the Social? Re-figuring the Territory of Government', *Economy and Society*, Vol. 25, No. 3, pp. 327–56.

Russell, A. (1998) 'Diamonds, Diplomacy and Dogs of War', *Electronic Telegraph*, Issue 1078, http://www.telegraph.co.uk

Securitas (1998) *Annual Report 1998*, Stockholm: Securitas AB.

Shearing, C. (1992) 'The Relations between Public and Private Policing', in M. Tonry and N. Morris (eds), *Modern Policing: Policing, Crime and Justice: A Review of Research*, Vol. 15, Chicago: University of Chicago Press.

Shearing, C. D. and Stenning, P. C. (eds) (1987) *Private Policing*, Newbury Park CA: Sage.

Shearing, C. D. and Wood, J. (forthcoming) 'Reflections on the Governance of Security: A Normative Enquiry'.

Sheptycki, J. (1995) 'Transnational Policing and the Makings of a Postmodern State', *British Journal of Criminology*, Vol. 35, No. 4, pp. 613–35.

Sheptycki, J. W. E. (1996) 'Law Enforcement, Justice and Democracy in the Transnational Arena: Reflections on the War on Drugs', *International Journal of the Sociology of Law*, Vol. 24, No. 1, pp. 24–75.

South, N. (1988) *Policing for Profit*, London: Sage.

Storch, R. (1976) 'The Policeman as Domestic Missionary: Urban Discipline and Popular Culture in Northern England 1850–1880', *Journal of Social History*, Vol. 9, No. 4, pp. 481–509.

Tyco International Ltd (1998) *Annual Report 1997*.

Tyco International Ltd (1999) *Annual Report 1998*.

UK Business Park (1998) Company Search: Securicor http://www.ukbusinesspark.co.uk

UK Equities Direct (1996) *UK Equities Direct*, Hemmington Scott Publishers.

US House of Representatives (1991) *Oversight Hearings on Alyeska Covert Operations*, 4 November.

US News and World Report (1997) 'Private Companies Train Armies around the World', 8 February.

de Waard, J. (1999) 'The Private Security Industry in International Perspective', *European Journal on Criminal Policy and Research*, Vol. 7, No. 1, pp. 143–74.

Wackenhut Corporation (1998) *Annual Report 1997*.

Woolf, M. (1996) 'British Firms Cash in on Crime', *The Observer*, 14 July.

2 Transnational policing and human rights

A case study

Jean-Paul Brodeur

Introduction

Since Malcolm Anderson's pioneering work (Anderson 1989), there has been a growing awareness of the transnationalisation of policing, which is exemplified by the increasing body of research addressing various aspects of this development (Benyon et al. 1993; Fijnaut 1993; Nadelman 1993; Anderson et al. 1995; Harding et al. 1995; Joubert and Bevers 1996; Sheptycki 1997, 1998a and b, to quote a few significant examples). I have recently argued that the transnationalisation of policing implied a blurring of the distinction between 'high' and 'low policing' (see: Brodeur 1983 for a discussion of these concepts), since enforcing the law in the global context is dependent on the gathering and sharing of intelligence, the hallmark of high policing (Brodeur 1998). Anderson et al. (1995: chapter five) also stress that the partial integration of police, state security and military forces into one network was a feature of transnational policing. Another feature of high policing is its threatening character for the respect of the due process of law and of human rights. Hence, the coming of age of transnational high policing should prompt us to reassess the adequacy of the present structures of police accountability (McLaughlin 1992; Lustgarten and Leigh 1994; Gill 1994).

This chapter will examine issues surrounding the due process of law and constitutional (human or civil) rights in the context of transnational policing. These issues will be approached through the presentation and discussion of two momentous legal cases which involved transnational policing. These two cases occurred in Canada during the course of the 1990s and the consequences are being felt even as this book goes to print. The first case pertains to the Can $50 million lawsuit filed by former Prime Minister Brian Mulroney against the government of Canada, after it had alleged that he was involved in criminal activities.

These allegations were made in the context of a request to the Swiss authorities for access to banking records thought to be connected to Mr Mulroney. This request was sent by the Canadian Department of Justice to the Swiss judicial authorities and was leaked to the press. The second case concerns the successful prosecution for money laundering of Quebec Superior Court judge Robert Flahiff. The investigation that led to this prosecution also involved a request to the Swiss authorities for the disclosure of banking information. In both cases it was the same Canadian official who made these requests.

The chapter is divided into four parts, followed by conclusions. The first two parts are devoted to a presentation of the two cases. The third part will briefly compare the two cases and highlight their common features and differences. The final section will discuss the major human rights issues raised. In the conclusion, I present suggestions for enhancing police accountability in the context of transnational policing.

The case of the former Prime Minister of Canada, Mr Brian Mulroney[1]

My presentation of the facts of the Mulroney case is not comprehensive. I have selected only the features of the case which have the greatest relevance for understanding transnational policing. The features outlined here certainly do not exhaust the more general significance of this case, particularly in respect to politicisation. The facts are rather complex since they initially involve two threads of events, one thread unfolding in Europe and the other in Canada.

The context

Mr Brian Mulroney was elected Prime Minister of Canada at the head of the Progressive Conservative Party, in 1984. The Progressive Conservatives held power until their resounding defeat by the Liberals in the 1993 federal election. In 1985, Air Canada, which was a Crown corporation that the Tories intended to privatise, decided to renew its fleet of planes. Three aircraft companies bid for the huge contract, these being: Boeing, McDonell Douglas and the European consortium Airbus Industrie. Air Canada finally decided in 1988 to buy 34 Airbus A320 aircraft at the cost of $1.8 billion, no doubt causing bitter disappointment among officials in the other corporations. Shortly thereafter, rumours began to spread which suggested that politicians had been paid off by Airbus. These rumours were fuelled by the fact that

Mr Frank Moores had been appointed to the Air Canada board of directors by the Tory Transport Minister Don Mazankowski in March 1985. Mr Moores, a prominent Tory who was Premier of the province of Newfoundland for seven years in the 1970s, had been an early supporter of Mr Mulroney's quest for the leadership of the Progressive Conservative Party. In 1985 he had become a member of a highly successful Tory lobbying firm – Government Consultant International (GCI) – and was on friendly terms with the Prime Minister. His appointment to the Air Canada board of directors was the subject of persistent criticism and he resigned in September 1985. This is an important fact which all too often seems to have escaped the notice of the scandalmongers who spread rumours of wrongdoing after Air Canada's 1988 decision to purchase its new planes from Airbus. Be that as it may, the Royal Canadian Mounted Police (RCMP; in French, Gendarmerie Nationale du Canada, GNC) eventually received a complaint from a source which remains undisclosed and a unit within the Economic Crime Directorate subsequently initiated an investigation.[2] The investigation was only intermittently pursued between 1988 and 1991, after which it was shelved. It was briefly reactivated in 1993, after the Liberals had been elected, but it again came to nothing and was again put down.

Before describing how the inquiry came to be resurrected yet again, there is one further element of the context that is worth mentioning. It was pointed out frequently in the French-language press in Quebec that the vilification of Mr Mulroney (whose home province is Quebec) became a preoccupation in the media of English-speaking Canada (Leblanc 1997). Both during the tenure of Mr Mulroney and after the Progressive Conservatives' defeat in 1993, there was a spate of books that were extremely critical of Mr Mulroney and his government (Hoy 1987; Cameron 1989, 1994; Fife 1991; Palango 1994) and these were accompanied by a no less enthusiastic effort at exposé in the newspapers and on television. Particularly damaging were the books of Mr Palango and Ms Cameron. In close association with Rod Stamler, a former RCMP officer, Mr Palango baldly asserted that Prime Minister Mulroney had pressured Air Canada into paying a $5-million commission to the company of his friend Frank Moores as a consulting fee for the purchase of the Airbus planes, although there is no documentary evidence that Mr Moores' consulting firm had played a part in the transaction (Palango 1994: 248).[3] Even more damaging was Ms Cameron's second book, entitled *On the Take: Crime, Corruption and Greed in the Mulroney Years* (Cameron 1994). Although the book did not contain anything of substance about Mr Mulroney himself, his enlarged photograph adorned the jacket of the book, which became a best-seller in Canada. These books created a climate of opinion which eroded, probably to a significant although unquantifiable extent, any presumption of innocence on Mr Mulroney's behalf. They lent seeming credibility to any allegation of wrongdoing made against him, and members of the RCMP came to share in the credulity thus produced. Indeed, these books licensed the official use of language bordering on the slanderous with respect to Mr Mulroney.[4]

The resumption of the investigation

One transnational aspect of this case, albeit a rather contingent one, comes in the person of Mr Karlheinz Schreiber, a German-born international businessman resident in the Canadian province of Alberta for almost 20 years. Schreiber made a living looking after the interests of wealthy German families in Canada, most notably those of Franz-Josef Strauss. Strauss had been a prominent and controversial German politician. He was Premier of Bavaria from 1978 to 1988, after having served as West Germany's Minister of Defence and, later, of Finance. In 1985, Strauss was also the chairman of the supervisory board of Airbus Industrie and in this capacity he asked Schreiber to act as the Canadian agent for Airbus, through his own company International Aircraft Leasing (IAL). IAL was also involved in several other ventures in Canada. Schreiber's IAL and Frank Moores' GCI were alleged to have been paid handsome commissions in the purchase in 1986 of German helicopters by the Canadian Coastguard. While representing another German firm, Thyssen AG, Schreiber also tried to convince the Canadian federal government to subsidise the opening of a manufacturing plant in Nova Scotia. This Thyssen subsidiary, called Bear Head, was to produce light armoured vehicles to be sold to the Canadian Armed forces. The project was finally cancelled in 1992 by Prime Minister Mulroney himself.

Schreiber hired one Giorgio Pelossi as his accountant in 1986. Mr Pelossi apparently abused his functions at IAL and was fired by Mr Schreiber at the end of 1991. He then decided to blow the whistle on Mr Schreiber's business transactions and started to talk with the journalist Mathias von Blumencron of *Der Spiegel* in 1992. This German magazine was interested in Pelossi's story, because it implicated Mr Schreiber's boss, Mr Strauss, one of *Der Spiegel*'s political nemeses. Mr Pelossi provided *Der Spiegel* with several compromising documents implicating IAL for the receipt of payments totalling millions of Canadian dollars in 'commission' for the purchase of Airbus planes by

Air Canada. Since Mr Pelossi's revelations involved transnational business deals between European companies and the Canadian government, *Der Spiegel* contacted Mr Jock Ferguson, a researcher for *The Fifth Estate*, a Canadian television news series that specialised in investigative reporting. Mr Ferguson travelled to Germany, where von Blumencron shared with him the documents that he had obtained from Pelossi. More fatefully, Ferguson also met Pelossi. Pelossi told him that in 1986 he went to a branch of the Swiss Bank Corporation with Karlheinz Schreiber and Frank Moores and that they opened two numbered accounts – 34107 and 34117. The second of these accounts was given the code name 'Devon' – this happens to be the name of a street in Westmount (Quebec) where Brian Mulroney had bought a house in 1973. Furthermore, Mr Pelossi claimed that, in notes taken at the time, he had written that the initials 'B.M.' appeared beside the number of the Devon account on the bank manager's business card. Pelossi also told Ferguson that Schreiber had explained to him that this second account was to receive commissions paid to Brian Mulroney.[5] Enticed by the possibility of a good story, *Der Spiegel* and *The Fifth Estate* decided to go on digging. In March 1995, *Der Spiegel* published a first article on the commissions, totalling up to US $46 million, that Schreiber's IAL had received for the sale of Airbus planes to Air Canada, although IAL had played no part as Airbus's agent in this deal. In a second and even more damaging story, the German news magazine claimed that Mr Schreiber was not the only party to have benefited from suspicious commissions and that Mr Frank Moores and Mr Brian Mulroney had also shared in the loot.[6] These stories were rapidly picked up by the press of Montreal – *La Presse*, 19 March 1995 and *The Montreal Gazette*, 20 March 1995 – where Mr Mulroney and his family lived. On 28 March 1995, *The Fifth Estate* finally aired the findings of its inquiry in a programme during which Mr Pelossi was interviewed without his identity being revealed. Although conceding that there was no evidence that anybody with 'decision-making powers' – that is, someone within the Canadian government – had accepted any money, *The Fifth Estate* did assert that Mr Schreiber and Mr Frank Moores were involved in payments from Airbus Industrie. Furthermore, Mr Pelossi stated that two bank accounts had been opened in a Swiss bank in 1986, one of them being for Frank Moores and the other one for a Canadian politician, whom he did not name.

Although the RCMP had closed the file on the Airbus investigation in 1991 and again in 1993, after an attempt by the new Liberal Minister of Justice to revive it, it decided to resume the investigation after the *Fifth Estate* broadcast. Actually, according to Kaplan's chronology (Kaplan 1998: 337), the RCMP came into possession of the *Fifth Estate* documents in January 1995, that is, two months *before* the programme was aired. Sergeant Fraser Fiegenwald of the Commercial Crime Unit was the sole officer assigned to the case. He immediately set to work on the documents[7] but saw no need to interview Pelossi, who was then easily available. Sergeant Fiegenwald decided to broaden the scope of his inquiry and to add to the Airbus affair, the Bear Head project and the sale of German helicopters to the Coastguard. Schreiber was involved in both of these additional ventures and Moores in at least one of them.

The request and the leak

A treaty on Mutual Assistance in Criminal Matters (MLAT/SW) had been signed between Switzerland and Canada in Bern on 7 October 1993, but was not to be in force before 17 November 1995.[8] Before the treaty came into force, Swiss banking information had to be requested through an official letter sent to the Swiss legal authorities. All the requests were processed by the International Assistance Group (IAG) of the Department of Justice, a small unit headed by a lawyer named Kimberly Prost. Sergeant Fiegenwald submitted to Mrs Prost the first draft of his request between the end of June 1995 and the beginning of July. It was extensively revised to meet the requirements of Swiss law and was finally signed and sent to Switzerland by Mrs Prost on 29 September 1995. In processing this request involving a former Canadian Prime Minister, Mrs Prost consulted her immediate supervisor, William H. Corbett, and the matter was kept at their level. The letter requested the Swiss bank records of Moores, Mulroney and Schreiber, in particular the records for the two accounts opened in the presence of Mr Pelossi in 1986. It began by stating that the information was requested in 'relation to the investigation and prosecution of *alleged* violations of Canadian criminal law by Brian Mulroney and Frank Moores' (quoted in Kaplan 1998: 86, my emphasis). However, in later paragraphs the letter elided the language of allegation. As it became more blunt, the request for banking information was couched in language plainly asserting that the suspects had violated the criminal law and concluded thus:

> The above three cases demonstrate an ongoing scheme by Mr
> Mulroney, Mr Moores and Mr Schreiber to defraud the Canadian
> government of millions of dollars of public funds from the time

Mr Mulroney took office in September 1984, until he resigned in June 1993 . . . This investigation is of serious concern to the government of Canada as it involves criminal activity on the part of a former Prime Minister. Further investigation cannot be conducted by the RCMP until the information available in Switzerland is received. Any priority which could be placed on this request would be gratefully appreciated.

(Quoted in Kaplan 1998: 89)

On 26 October, the Swiss federal prosecutor, Carla del Ponte, acquiesced to the Canadian request in the main.[9] In compliance with Swiss banking law, Moores and Schreiber were notified of the Canadian request and received a copy of the letter sent by Prost. As it was quickly found that Mr Mulroney had neither bank account nor safety deposit box in Switzerland, he was not himself notified of the Canadian request. However, Schreiber informed Mulroney about the allegations of his involvement in a series of serious illicit financial transactions through a third party. Mulroney in turn contacted Schreiber and convinced him to forward an English translation of the German version of the Prost letter. Schreiber sent Mulroney an English translation that had been made for his Canadian lawyer, Robert Hladun, by his Swiss legal counsel (Blum and Partners).

On 2 November, just over a month from the drafting of the letter of request to Swiss authorities, Mr Mulroney retained the services of lawyer Roger Tassé, a former deputy minister at the Department of Justice. Tassé offered full co-operation with the RCMP in its investigation on the condition that the Prost letter be withdrawn and replaced by a less accusatory one. Mulroney's offer of co-operation was rejected by Sergeant Fiegenwald on 17 November. In the meantime, it became obvious that the story was being leaked to the press. Although Mr Tassé was acting confidentially on behalf of Brian Mulroney, he was being sought by Stevie Cameron, Mr Mulroney's chief nemesis, who wanted to ask about his secret meetings with the RCMP and justice department officials. Ms Cameron evidently had a good source of information in government. Meanwhile, the Canadian request for banking information was generating stories on Swiss television, by the Agence Française de Presse and, increasingly, by the local media in Quebec. It was only a matter of days before the full content of the Prost letter was published in the press.

This finally came to pass on 18 November, one day after the offer from Mr Mulroney to co-operate with the RCMP investigation had been refused. The story was published in the Canadian *Financial Post* under the headline 'Justice seeks evidence on Mulroney, Moores' (Mathias 1995a) but it actually only quoted small parts of the letter's conclusion. On the same day, Mr Mulroney's lawyers announced in a press conference that he was suing the RCMP and the Government of Canada for $50 million ($25 million for damages to Mr Mulroney's reputation and $25 million for punitive damages, which would be given to charity). The version of the Canadian request to Switzerland that the *Financial Post* disclosed was the English translation from the German originally provided to Mr Schreiber by his Swiss lawyers. It was thus alleged that, since it was Schreiber who had sent a copy of this translation to Mr Mulroney, it was he (Schreiber) who had leaked the letter to the press. The leak was said to be an attempt to circumvent a threatening criminal investigation by creating the possibility of a libel action. However, the *Post* reporter, Mr Philip Mathias, continues to deny that Mr Mulroney had leaked the letter to him.

The libel lawsuit and its settlement

This part of the case lasted from 18 November 1995 to 6 January 1997. It was extensively reported in the Canadian (especially English-language) media, the preliminary procedures for the civil trial having been held in public. A full account of this falls outside the scope of this chapter, but two things must be mentioned for the purposes of the discussion to come. First, in March 1996, Karlheinz Schreiber initiated proceedings in the Federal Court of Canada, claiming that the request sent by the Department of Justice to Switzerland should have received prior judicial authorisation in Canada and was thus sent in violation of his constitutional rights. We shall discuss these proceedings and their outcome in detail shortly. Second, the case was finally prevented from going to court because of a chance happening. A few days before the opening of the trial, the chief government lawyer learned that RCMP Sergeant Fiegenwald had leaked information to reporter Stevie Cameron early on in the case naming Mr Mulroney as 'the Canadian politician' mentioned in the Prost letter. As the government's defence was essentially based on the claim that every official involved in this case had acted properly and in good faith, it collapsed and the government felt compelled to settle the case before the trial began, although it had previously determined to fight the case in court (Ha et al. 1997). According to the settlement, the government of Canada acknowledged that any conclusions of wrongdoing by the former Prime Minister were – and are – unjustified; it apologised to Mr Mulroney and his family and accepted to pay all of Mr Mulroney's legal fees, which were in excess of $2 million.[10] However, Mr Mulroney could not obtain the closing of the investigation, which was reopened in August 1999.[11] It was widely perceived in the press that the government's apologies were made with so little conviction that they added insult to injury. As of this writing, the person who signed the letter, Mrs Kimberly Prost, remains in her post in the IAG at the Canadian Department of Justice and is still performing the same duties.

The case of Superior Court Judge Robert Flahiff

My presentation of this case will be shorter than the previous one, as the investigation and prosecution of Judge Robert Flahiff was successful and relatively uneventful, despite its high media profile. The chronology of events presented here is retrospective and has been reconstructed in the light of what was later learned during the police investigation. I have relied on court documents, interviews and my own file of press reports for the description of this case.

The context

Mr Robert Flahiff was a practising criminal lawyer from 1975 to 1993, at which time he was appointed to the Superior Court of the province of Quebec. From 1986 to approximately 1990, he represented in various capacities Mr Paul Larue, who was trafficking in cocaine. Paul Larue was a fairly big-time trafficker and made at least $10 million from 1976 to 1986. Between 1986 and 1988, the relationship between Flahiff and his client Larue did not involve the outright commission of crimes by the lawyer but he became progressively more embroiled into the illegal activities of his client. In June 1986, he was paid $25,000 by Paul Larue to recuperate $350,000 seized by the American customs when one of his accomplices attempted to enter the US to deliver this money to Colombian drug traffickers. In August 1987, he was paid $40,000 to make sure that another of Larue's accomplices, who had been accused of murdering his wife, would not reveal anything on the drug-trafficking organisation in the course of his prosecution. During those years, Larue was having serious problems with his income tax reports and paid $300,000 to another lawyer, Richard Blanchette, for providing him with false documents which showed that his income was legal. Flahiff convinced Larue that he was paying Blanchette too much and offered to solve his income tax problems for $150,000 dollars. Larue accepted this offer and Flahiff went into partnership with another lawyer, Gérald Lavoie, to take care of Larue's income tax problems.

Money laundering

Flahiff later offered to help Larue by investing his drug profits in Switzerland, providing that the sums to be invested were substantial – $500,000 for each venture. Larue agreed to invest more than Can $2 million. From 1988 to 1991, Flahiff and his accomplice Lavoie laundered close to one million dollars for Larue. The scheme operated in the following way. Flahiff would buy large drafts from the Bank of Montreal and deliver them personally to a Swiss broker, Mr Kurt Gafner of the firm Geremant, who then invested the money in various securities. The money was invested through the Swiss bank Ferrier Lullin for the Altor Trading Corporation, which at the time was a front for the sole benefit of Paul Larue. After a period of time, the money would be channelled back to Montreal via complicated circuits involving banking institutions in the Caribbean. Flahiff and Lavoie received a commission of 5 to 10 per cent for the monies thus laundered, plus travelling expenses. In 1990, Flahiff was apparently pressing Larue to invest more money but the latter became suspicious and put an end to his dealings with Flahiff and Lavoie in 1991. In January 1993, Robert Flahiff was appointed to the bench of the Superior Court of Quebec. He has not been accused of criminal activities perpetrated after he became a judge.

The investigation

On 21 March 1993, Paul Larue was arrested and prosecuted in the US for drug trafficking. He was eventually sentenced to 17 years in a Florida penitentiary subsequent to which he offered his co-operation to the US and Canadian authorities in the hope of having his sentence reduced. He was interviewed by Sergeant Detective McGarr of the Montreal City Police, at which time he disclosed the part that the lawyers Flahiff and Lavoie had played in laundering the profits he had made from drug trafficking. Sergeant McGarr filed a report of the interview but did not pursue the investigation further because he believed that Paul Larue would not make a credible witness in the absence of corroborating evidence. In 1994, McGarr's report implicating Flahiff resurfaced in the trial of Mr Paulin Bolduc, another former accomplice of Larue. The allegations against Judge Flahiff circulated among the persons attending the trial, which was held in the Quebec city of Sherbrooke,[12] and there was consequently no way of avoiding the resumption of the investigation, which was undertaken by the RCMP. In April 1994, the RCMP investigator Gilles Charette interviewed Larue in prison in Florida and obtained from him a signed declaration implicating Robert Flahiff in money laundering, when he was his lawyer. Larue also volunteered to testify against Flahiff in exchange for a financial reward for himself and his wife. More decisively, however, Charette was given Larue's electronic diary by the Florida authorities. Larue had provided Charette with the access code to the secret part of the diary, which was discovered to contain information on the money-laundering operation. It appeared to show that Flahiff took care of the banking transactions to launder the money, while Lavoie took care of the income tax side. The diary also yielded the name of the Swiss broker, Kurt Gafner, an address and a telephone number in Switzerland, and it also listed two phone numbers for Robert Flahiff. Through the IAG, and the offices of Mrs Prost, the RCMP made a request for the bank records of Paul Larue and of all the transactions made on behalf of Altor trading.[13] While this first request was made when the MLAT between Switzerland and Canada was not yet in force, the RCMP was provided with more than 160 documents by the Swiss.

The prosecution

Following the reception of these documents, Larue was interviewed again by two investigators – one from the RCMP and the other from the Quebec provincial police – and various searches and seizures were also conducted in the Montreal area. It was concluded that the evidence was quite possibly strong enough to warrant the prosecution of Robert Flahiff, even though he was a Superior Court Judge. The legal authorities then made the critical decision of appointing Mr Bruno Pateras, a legal expert on economic crime, as special prosecutor for this case. Counsel Pateras was put in charge of the prosecution on 16 December 1996.[14] Because of the crucial nature of this prosecution, Bruno Pateras decided that he would review the whole police inquiry. Using the MLAT/SW that had since come into force, he travelled with two Canadian investigators to Switzerland, where he had all the documents that he intended to use as evidence officially authenticated, in order for them to be admissible in a Canadian court. Upon a Swiss magistrate's order, the broker Kurt Gafner was interviewed by a team comprising the Swiss magistrate, Mr Pateras, as well as Swiss and Canadian investigators. At the end of this new investigation, the special prosecutor decided to charge Judge Flahiff with several counts relating to three different offences, which together amounted to the laundering of the profits of criminal activities. Judge Flahiff was eventually found guilty of all three charges in January 1999 and sentenced on 6 February of that year to three years of incarceration for each offence, to be served concurrently. As of this writing he is pursuing an appeal of both the verdict and the sentence.

Common features and differences

There are many common features between these two cases at the level of facts. Both occurred during the same period of time (the mid- to late 1990s) and involved transnational information exchange between the same two countries (Canada and Switzerland). The RCMP was involved in both investigations and, interestingly, the legal authorities who handled the official correspondence regarding requests for information were the same in both instances (Kimberly Prost for Canada and Carla del Ponte for Switzerland).[15] Although the crimes alleged were rather different – secret commissions in the Mulroney affair and drug money laundering in the Flahiff case – they both belong to the class of crimes labelled transnational economic crime. In both instances, the persons implicated either held a public office or were connected to a high-ranking public official: Brian Mulroney is a former Canadian Prime Minister; Frank Moores was once a provincial Premier; Karlheinz Schreiber worked for Franz-Josef Strauss and was a partner of Frank Moores; and Robert Flahiff was a Quebec Superior Court judge. The status of these individuals thus ensured that these cases would have a high media profile. In both instances the persons investigated were brought into the limelight by informants who had motivations other than the public good: Giorgio Pelossi wanted revenge against Karlheinz Schreiber who had fired him and Paul Larue was a convicted felon ready to trade incriminating information against former accomplices for a reduction of sentence. With respect to the investigative process, two common features should be emphasised. In both cases the initial investigation was dropped and reactivated: this occurred several times in the Mulroney affair and at least once in the Flahiff case. Finally, and perhaps most importantly, both cases required the access to information that was not already in the hands of any police force: the RCMP was not asking for Swiss *police* information but for Swiss *banking* information. Transnational policing is a process which involves much greater complexity when it goes beyond transactions between two police forces, whether these transactions are pursued 'face to face' or more formally.

There are many circumstantial differences between the two cases, which are not significant for the purposes of this paper (e.g. in the

Mulroney affair, allegations were made against three persons, whereas Judge Flahiff was the only defendant in his case; one police informant was a convicted felon (Larue), whereas the other (Pelossi) blew the whistle in the media and was neither charged nor convicted of a crime). One difference needs to be stressed however. Robert Flahiff was not accused of having abused his power as a judge for his own criminal benefit since his dealings with Larue were finished when he was appointed judge, but in the case involving Brian Mulroney the most damning allegation made was that he had abused the office of Prime Minister. This accounts for the high politicisation of his case.

However, the truly significant differences concern process. First, in the Mulroney case, the proceedings were apparently stopped at their initial stage, that is, the request for banking information sent to Switzerland; in the case of Judge Flahiff, the whole process successfully unfolded for the government, the investigation leading to prosecution and to a criminal conviction. Second, there were no allegations of a violation of human rights[16] in the Flahiff case, where the basic facts of the case were agreed by both the defence and the prosecution.[17] In the Mulroney case, not only were the allegations resisted, they resulted in several court proceedings. We shall now examine what generated these differences.

Discussion

What is it that went wrong in the Mulroney affair, as compared to everything that went right in the Flahiff case? To answer this question, we shall contrast the two cases from their incipient stages.

The first issue actually points to shared features of the two cases under discussion. It is the discretion enjoyed by the police in deciding to open, to close and to reactivate an investigation. The Airbus investigation was (re)activated and dropped in 1988, 1993, 1995; it was activated again in August 1999. The allegations of Paul Larue against Judge Flahiff were not at first investigated by the municipal police of Montreal, who believed he would not make a credible witness. The lesson is that police discretion not to invoke the law is largely unfettered (Goldstein 1960) as long as the incriminating allegations are not made in a public forum. When low-visibility decisions become high-visibility decisions the nature of police discretion changes. Thus, when the allegations of Paul Larue against Judge Flahiff resurfaced in a public trial, they were thoroughly investigated and subsequently validated. When the allegations of Mr Pelossi against an 'unnamed Canadian politician' were aired on the CBC's *Fifth Estate* programme which was broadcast in January 1995, the investigation resumed. However, in contrast with Mr Larue who himself used Mr Flahiff to launder his money, Mr Pelossi never was in contact with Mr Mulroney and his allegations were little more than hearsay.[18] The simple fact that these allegations were publicised by the media, however unsubstantiated they were, triggered a reopening of the RCMP investigation. Indeed, a videotape of *The Fifth Estate* and copies of the articles published in *Der Spiegel* were appended to the Canadian request to the Swiss authorities as justifications for it.

A second issue is whether the policing authorities who request information from a foreign country are fully aware of its laws and regulations (cf. Sheptycki 1996, 1998c). The lack of such knowledge may not only jeopardise a police investigation, but may also cause grievous harm to a person's reputation. Both of these things happened in the Mulroney affair.[19] What initially prompted Mr Mulroney to act successfully against the Canadian government was that he obtained, through Mr Schreiber, a copy of the Canadian request to the Swiss authorities, which implicated him. Neither the low-ranking police officers nor the junior civil servant in charge of the case knew that copies of their request would start to circulate nor could they have foreseen that they would end up in the Canadian press through a leak.[20] This confirms the need to improve mutual legal knowledge among the partners in transnational policing which has been stressed by Joubert and Bevers (1996: 539).

With regard to process, there are two important differences between the Mulroney affair and the Flahiff case: first, the degree of justification for the respective information requests sent to Switzerland and, second, the fact that the request involving Mr Mulroney was leaked to the press. I shall discuss both of these differences in turn. The request for information sent in the course of the Flahiff investigation was based on solid grounds. What was found in Larue's electronic diary provided strong and detailed corroboration of his declarations to the police and fully warranted the Canadian requests – there were two – to the Swiss authorities for financial information. Notwithstanding that Mr Mulroney claimed during the preliminary stages of his lawsuit that the request sent to Switzerland contained 29 affirmations of fact that were false (quoted in Kaplan 1998: 186) and that the Canadian government later apologised to Mr Mulroney for the language used in this request, there is clear evidence that much was wrong with the letter sent by Kimberly Prost on 29 September 1995. Some weeks later, when the media was awash with rumours, Mrs Prost sent another letter to her Swiss counterpart, Mr Pascal Gossin, which stressed the need for the request to be kept confidential. In that second letter she expressed concern that out-of-context disclosure of the request, or parts thereof, could be damaging to both the investigation and the reputation of the persons it involved.[21] It is possible to infer that the Swiss authorities understood that the letter of request contained allegations and that no conclusion had yet been reached on the guilt or innocence of the persons under investigation. However, if the content of the first letter had been sufficiently grounded in fact and was written in language which preserved the subject's presumption of innocence no second letter would have been necessary.

Why was the first letter sent in its controversial formulation and even at all? There are obvious answers to this question. First, such requests very often make short shrift of the presumption of innocence: the conflating of hypothetical allegations and factual assertions is in the nature of their style. Second, the request was handled by low-ranking officers, at first unaware of the implications of their action.[22] However, the issue was raised as a result of a legal action initiated by Karlheinz Schreiber, one of Mr Mulroney's 'co-defendants'. The issue raised by Mr Schreiber is neatly summarised by the Supreme Court of Canada, which ultimately decided the case:

> Was the Canadian standard for the issuance of a search warrant required to be satisfied before the Minister of Justice and Attorney General of Canada submitted the Letter of Request asking Swiss authorities to search for and seize the Plaintiff's [now the respondent's] banking documents and records?

In other words, Mr Schreiber's lawyer claimed that the RCMP should have applied for a search warrant from a Canadian judge before sending its request to Switzerland through a Justice Department official. The Supreme Court of Canada ultimately rejected this claim and answered the question in the negative (Schreiber v. Canada [1998] 1 R.C.S.). The legal history of this case reveals, however, that the issue is far from settled. Mr Schreiber won in the Federal Court, Trial Division ([1996] 3 F.C. 931). When the case was appealed by the government, he also won in the Federal Court of Appeal ([1997] 2 F.C. 176), with one of the three judges dissenting. This dissent opened the way for a last appeal before the Supreme Court, which decided against Mr Schreiber. However, the ruling of the seven Supreme Court judges was far from unanimous. Not only did two judges express a strong dissent, but even the five judges who ruled that the Canadian authorities were not required to apply for a judicial warrant in order to send a request for secret banking information to Switzerland substantially disagreed on the reasons supporting their position.

Why was the Canadian request assented to by the Swiss authorities? Although the MLAT/SW signed on 7 October 1993 was to be in force only on 17 November, a common political will to facilitate mutual legal assistance prevailed at the time between Switzerland and Canada. The Canadian request originally drafted by Sergeant Fiegenwald of the RCMP was six pages long. As has been shown, it was transmitted to the Department of Justice at the end of July 1995 and sent to Switzerland two months later, on 29 September. By then, its length had grown to eleven single-spaced pages and its wording was much more accusatory than in the original RCMP draft. It is on public record that there were several drafts of this letter, Mr Mulroney's lawyers having obtained parts of an earlier sketch of the final letter. It was claimed by Mr Schreiber's lawyer that the letter had received pre-approval from the Swiss authority before being sent (Kaplan 1998: 223), which suggests that the Swiss authorities reviewed earlier versions of the request which they finally accepted. It has been reported that Mrs Prost described the role of the IAG as merely that of a mailbox through which the RCMP and other police forces send their requests for assistance in criminal matters to foreign countries, and that she did so in a meeting with Mr Roger Tassé, the first lawyer who was retained by Mr Mulroney (Kaplan 1998: 100).[23] Regardless of her precise form of words, her Department's position was later articulated by a legal expert hired by the Canadian government: Mrs Prost had an obligation not to interfere with the investigation conducted by the police but her job was to provide them with advice on how to comply with the legal requirements of the foreign countries from which they requested information (p. 241). I would want to argue that this hands-off policy in respect to police investigation only begets hands-on interference with citizens' rights. It exemplifies the kind of skewed neutrality that one too often finds in the operation of criminal justice.

The second important difference between the Mulroney and the Flahiff cases with regard to how things proceeded is that there was no leak in the latter case. Legal opinions are still very divided in Canada with respect to what went wrong in the Mulroney affair, but many believe that the only fault was the leaking of the letter supporting the Canadian request. Are such leaks threatening to be more frequent in the context of transnational policing? As we saw, it was in Germany where *Der Spiegel* linked the name of Mr Mulroney to the Airbus transaction. Since suing a news media source operating in another country for libel is fraught with serious difficulties, the possibility of a civil lawsuit is a weaker deterrent of defamation in a transnational context than it is in respect to the national press. Hence, leaks and innuendoes may become more frequent in the global context of transnational policing. This underlines the need to control police discretion in the use of media allegations which, on their own, should not justify launching a transnational police investigation.

The opposite of leaking information is withholding it. The Canadian government systematically objected to the disclosure of information vital to the Mulroney and Schreiber defences on the grounds that it would undermine commitments to foreign countries which had agreed to provide legal assistance and thus would jeopardise future international co-operation in criminal matters. Thus 'international trust' seems to provide a legal justification for secrecy in transnational law enforcement in much the same way that the notion of 'national security' has in the more traditional (i.e. national) law enforcement setting (Sallot 1997).

Finally, there is one last crucial difference between the Mulroney and the Flahiff cases. Notwithstanding rumours of political interference that were never substantiated, the case which implicated Mulroney, Moores and Schreiber was always steered by low-level officials, within both the RCMP and the Department of Justice. The case against Flahiff was undertaken by more senior personnel. Mr Bruno Pateras, a highly respected practising lawyer in the field of economic crime, was called in as soon as it appeared that the evidence gathered against Judge Flahiff by the RCMP could warrant prosecution. To all practical purposes, Mr Pateras assumed, in a common law context, the role of a French *juge d'instruction*.[24] Because of the high stakes of this prosecution against a Superior Court judge, he took up again, as we saw, the police investigation in all of its steps and travelled to Switzerland with two police investigators. The assistance of the Swiss authorities was requested a second time, through the MLAT/SW, which had come into force. Although the MLAT between Switzerland and Canada spells out more explicitly the procedure for obtaining legal assistance from Switzerland, there was no truly significant difference between making a request for legal assistance before the coming into force of this treaty and after. Mr Pateras's main concern was to make sure that the evidence was overwhelming and that there would be no objection to its admissibility in court. His caution in this regard is a matter of public record, indeed he has stated that 'one does not accuse a judge frivolously' (*On n'accuse pas un juge à la légère*). Astonishingly enough, it would seem that a former Prime Minister can be treated in the most cavalier fashion in circumstances not much different. It must be stressed that Mr Pateras was put in charge of the proceedings after the initial phase of the police investigation had been successfully completed. The Mulroney investigation has not yet moved beyond this stage and it is doubtful that it ever will.

Conclusion

The police must go through government channels such as the IAG when the information that they seek lies outside the scope of available criminal intelligence. Transnational policing thus entails the establishment of two kinds of relationships: those between police forces of different countries (that is: between sub-state agencies) and relationships between their respective governments (that is: intergovernmental ones). This paper has illuminated the latter type of interaction, which has tended to receive less attention in the literature on transnational policing than has the former. One certain point comes out of the analysis of these cases and that is, with due regard to the increased visibility of corruption at the highest levels of the global polity, policing is going to be increasingly dependent on, involved with, and implicated in, transnational relations between governments and their personnel.

What ultimately spelled success in the Flahiff prosecution and failure in the aborted Mulroney investigation was the issue of control. The Mulroney 'affair' would never have taken off if confidentiality had been respected during the investigation and, connectedly, if the successive drafts of the request had been properly supervised. In the Flahiff case, similar problems occurred, but on a much more limited scale, when Mr Flahiff's name unexpectedly surfaced in court proceedings. When Mr Pateras took charge, he made sure that they did not happen again, which illustrates that scrupulous management of such cases is both necessary and possible.

Controlling police actions and making police agencies accountable are among the oldest questions raised by the defence of human rights. Because of its inter-institutional complexity, transnational policing seems to be a return to much older practices, when there was little control and accountability. While it is hindered by bureaucratic 'red tape', and perhaps *because* it is, transnational policing strives for results rather than propriety; in the language of criminal jurisprudence, for crime control rather than due process. For instance, MLATs revert to the old dichotomy between political and common crimes as a way of limiting the obligation to provide mutual assistance; common crimes are open to police co-operation but political deviance is not. This is not adequate protection. Keeping fundamental rights from being drowned by the undertow of police pragmatism is a necessary step in promoting a balance between efficiency and due process.

In order to achieve this result, the fountainhead of police accountability has to be reinvented. The cases which we have discussed tend to show that once a request has been cleared in the requesting country it will be met by the foreign authorities to whom it is addressed, particularly if there is an MLAT between the two countries involved. Hence, the country from which the request originates should be the place to begin setting up formal structures of control specially intended for transnational policing. Over time, it is to be hoped that international instruments such as the Universal Declaration of Human Rights or the European Convention on Human Rights will come to play a bigger part in such monitoring, but this will require the efficient and effective functioning of supra-national bodies like the European Court of Human Rights, or indeed an International Criminal Court. Over the longer term, it is to be hoped that transnational proceedings in criminal matters will result in a cross-fertilisation of the various national legal traditions. In this respect, reviewing the role of magistrates (or of prosecutors) in the oversight of police investigations against the background of their role as *juge d'instruction* in the inquisitorial system may yield particularly interesting results.

Notes

1 My presentation of the Mulroney case owes much to the recent book on this affair by William Kaplan, Professor of Law at the University of Ottawa (Kaplan 1998). Readers should be informed that Professor Kaplan approached Mr Mulroney in 1996 with a proposal to write a book on the then-pending lawsuit against the federal government. After the settlement of that suit, the former Prime Minister accepted the offer to participate in the project. Mr Kaplan was reportedly given full access to Mr Mulroney, his team and their files in researching the book. The Canadian Government was much less forthcoming and so it can fairly be said that Mr Kaplan's book represents the Mulroney version of these events much more than that of the government. Unfortunately, access to government papers related to this case may never be granted for 'security reasons'. Having followed this case from its beginning, I therefore have also relied on my own media files, on legal documents that can be found in the public domain, and on personal interviews. Kaplan's book provided a guide to the essential facts of what was, and still remains, a complicated case. In what follows all matters of interpretation are my own, unless otherwise specified.

2 The RCMP is the federal police force of Canada. It undertakes general police duties in a number of provincial jurisdictions, but also offers spe-

cialist investigative capacities for certain types of crime, notably economic crime (including money laundering) and drug trafficking. However, it is important to note that the RCMP does not exercise a monopoly over the investigation of these crimes, which can also be undertaken by provincial and municipal police forces (for a schematic overview of the Canadian police system which remains reasonably accurate despite some organisational changes, see Mawby 1990).

3 Mr Palango does not provide a source for his assertion. Interestingly, there was no public reaction from Mr Mulroney to the publication of the book while, by reading between the lines, one might infer a deep resentment against Mr Mulroney and his government within certain elements of the RCMP.

4 In one article Philip Mathias of the Canadian *Financial Post* observed that Mr Mulroney would have to overcome the barrier of his already 'greatly diminished' reputation in order to win his civil suit for libel against the government (Mathias 1995b: 5).

5 In a 1995 interview with reporter Philip Mathias of *The Financial Post*, Frank Moores said that this second account had been established for his wife – Beth Moores, hence the 'B.M.' besides the account number – and that the code 'Devon' was given by him to the account, because his parents came from Devon. The account was closed in 1990 and the bank records that were published by Mathias in the *Post* with his story show that no important sum of money was ever placed in this account. See Kaplan 1998: 150.

6 *Der Spiegel* was quite specific in its allegations. The headline of the article was 'An account with a code-name' (*Konto mit Code-Wort*), thus explicitly referring to the account with the code-name 'Devon', which pointed to Mr Mulroney, who was mentioned by name in the article as a close friend of Frank Moores. See *Der Spiegel*, 1995, No. 14, in the '*Wirtschaft*' section.

7 There are questions as to how the *Fifth Estate* file came into the hands of the RCMP. Kaplan states that 'a journalist' or 'the press' passed these documents to the RCMP in violation of journalistic ethics, but does not identify any person by name (Kaplan 1998: 66, 328, 337). He also acknowledges that David Studer, the executive producer of *The Fifth Estate*, has denied that the documents were provided by his team (p. 148). What cannot be denied is that the RCMP came into possession of these documents originally transmitted by Pelossi to the press.

8 For the text of this treaty, see *Canada Gazette Part I*, 9 December 1995. These treaties are governed by the Mutual Legal Assistance in Criminal Matters Act, R.S.C. c. 30 (4th Supp.).

9 Mrs del Ponte became Prosecutor for the International Criminal Tribunal created in relation to the crimes committed in former Yugoslavia and in Kosovo, replacing the Canadian Louise Arbour at the end of 1999.

10 For the full text of the settlement see *The Globe and Mail*, 7 January 1997, p. A 4.

11 See *The Globe and Mail*, 18 August 1999, pp. 1 and A6. Also see the issues of *The Globe and Mail, The National Post, The Montreal Gazette* and of the Montreal French daily *La Presse* on the following day. Although the RCMP is proceeding on the basis of the September 1995 request for information on the bank records of Brian Mulroney, Frank Moores and

Karlheinz Schreiber, it seems that the main target of the inquiry is Mr Schreiber, who is also under investigation by the German police. However, as is always the case when trying to write the history of the present, the situation remains fluid; the front page headline of *The National Post* for 3 September 1999 revealed that: 'Swiss find no link to Mulroney in accounts' (Mathias, 1999). According to the news story: 'A letter sent last week by Swiss authorities to Brian Mulroney states that there is nothing to link the former prime minister with Swiss bank accounts held by German business-man Karlheinz Schreiber, the man at the center of the Airbus affair. In a letter sent on 23 August to Mr Mulroney's lawyers at McCarthy Tetreault in Montreal, Andreas Huber-Schlatter, secretary general of the Swiss Federal Department of Justice and Police, said: "Please note that none of the bank records so far produced or yet to be produced involve accounts of Mr Mulroney."' (Mathias, 1999).

12 The presiding judge at Bolduc's trial issued an order for the allegations against his fellow judge Flahiff not to be published in the press. But the cat was out of the bag, even if it was not allowed to roam the streets. Too many persons knew of the allegations against Flahiff for them to be kept secret.

13 NB: Mrs Prost is the same Department of Justice official who signed the request for the banking records of Messrs Moores, Mulroney and Schreiber, on 29 September 1995.

14 Coincidentally, Mr Bruno Pateras also represented the government of Canada from April 1996 to January 1997 in the attempts to reach an out-of-court settlement with Mr Mulroney in his libel lawsuit.

15 For a very brief period of time Mr Bruno Pateras was involved in both cases – from 16 December 1996 to 6 January 1997. In both instances, he was representing the government side. This short overlap was wholly co-incidental.

16 To be fully precise, it must be said that Judge Flahiff asked for a stay of proceedings on the basis of a violation of Article 11d of The Canadian Charter of Rights and Freedoms, which guarantees that a person will be judged by a tribunal that is impartial and independent. Financial security being in Canada a fundamental character of judicial independence, Judge Flahiff claimed that the Court of Quebec was not independent because the Quebec government had not followed the recommendations of a committee appointed to review the salary of the court judges. Not only was this motion rejected by the Court – [1999] R.J.Q. 877–883 – but it has no bearing on any issue of human rights in the context of transnational policing.

17 Judge Flahiff pleaded that there was no proof that the monies he invested for Paul Larue were the profit of drug trafficking and that, even if this was the case, he did not know about it. No witnesses were heard for the defence at the trial which proceeded in this regard on the basis of affidavits and certified documents. However, the prosecution did call witnesses to the stand.

18 Pelossi did give *Der Spiegel* documents implying that Karlheinz Schreiber had received commissions from Airbus to secure the sale of its planes to Air Canada. However, as far as we know, none of these documents remotely implicated Mr Mulroney in the scheme.

19 In the Flahiff case, the banking records on which information was requested were connected to Paul Larue, who fully agreed to the request. Irrespective of whether or not Mr Mulroney was served notice of the request for information from Swiss authorities, its content filtered out during the court proceedings.
20 Sergeant Fiegenwald was actually leaking information to Ms Stevie Cameron. However, she never used this information to publish the scoop that Mr Mulroney was the politician named in the request.
21 This letter was also leaked to the press and part of it is quoted in Kaplan (1998: 119).
22 It was often alleged in Canada that the request was a political vendetta directed from higher up against Mr Mulroney. I do not discuss this aspect of the case for which there is no hard evidence and which, in any case, holds no immediate lessons for understanding transnational policing.
23 In a public 'statement of assumed facts', the Canadian government later denied that Mrs Prost had ever described the role of her unit as that of a mailbox. However, Mr Tassé, who was a deputy minister for two government departments for thirteen years (1972–85), is a highly credible witness, even if he was representing Mr Mulroney at the time.
24 I made this suggestion to Mr Pateras in the course of an interview and he did not disagree with it.

References

Alain, M. (1999) *The Trapezists and the Ground Crew*, Research Report, Montréal: Centre International de Criminologie Comparée, Université de Montréal.
Anderson, M. (1989) *Policing the World*, Oxford: Clarendon Press.
Anderson, M., den Boer, M., Cullen, P., Gilmore, W., Raab, C. and Walker, N. (1995) *Policing the European Union: Theory, Law and Practice*, Oxford: Clarendon Press.
Benyon, J., Turnbull, L., Willis, A., Woodward, R. and Beck, A. (1993) *Police Cooperation in Europe: An Investigation*, Leicester: University of Leicester, Centre for the Study of Public Order.
Brodeur, J.-P. (1983) 'High Policing and Low Policing: Remarks about the Policing of Political Activities', *Social Problems*, Vol. 30, No. 5, pp. 507–20.
Brodeur, J.-P. (1998) 'The Globalization of Security and Intelligence Agencies', paper presented at the seminar 'Security and Intelligence Services: Common Structures, Common Dangers?', University of Gotheborg, Sweden. Forthcoming in a book to be published by Frank Cass, London (L. Lustgarten and D. Tollbörg, eds).
Brodeur, J.-P. (1999) 'Cops and Spooks', *Police Practice and Research*, Vol. 1, No. 3, pp. 1–24.
Cameron, S. (1989) *Ottawa Inside Out: Power, Prestige and Scandal in the Nation's Capital*, Toronto: Key Porter.
Cameron, S. (1994) *On the Take: Crime, Corruption and Greed in the Mulroney Years*, Toronto: Macfarlane Walter and Ross.

Fife, R. (1991) *A Capital Scandal*, Toronto: Key Porter.

Fijnaut, C. (ed.) (1993) *The Internationalization of Police Cooperation in Western Europe*, Deventer: Kluwer Law and Taxation Publishers.

Gill, P. (1994) *Policing Politics: Security Intelligence and the Liberal Democratic State*, London: Frank Cass.

Globe and Mail, 'The Settlement', 7 January 1997, p. A4.

Goldstein, J. (1960) 'Police Discretion not to Invoke the Criminal Process: Low Visibility Decisions in the Administration of Justice', *Yale Law Journal*, Vol. 69, pp. 543–94.

Ha, Tu Thanh, Windsor, H., Sallot, J. (1997) 'Leak Helped Sink Airbus Defence', *Globe and Mail*, 7 January 1997, pp. 1 and A6.

Harding, C., Fennell, P., Jörg, N. and Swart, B. (eds) (1995) *Criminal Justice in Europe: A Comparative Study*, Oxford: Clarendon Press.

Hoy, C. (1987) *Friends in High Places*, Toronto: Key Porter.

Joubert, C. and Bevers, H. (1996) *Schengen Investigated: A Comparative Interpretation of the Schengen Provisions on International Police Cooperation in the Light of the European Convention on Human Rights*, The Hague: Kluwer Law International.

Kaplan, W. (1998) *Presumed Guilty: Brian Mulroney, the Airbus Affair, and the Government of Canada*, Toronto: McClelland and Stewart.

Leblanc, G. (1997) 'Une Mystérieuse Animosité Viscérale', *La Presse*, 11 January, p. B7.

Lustgarten, L. and Leigh, I. (1994) *In from the Cold: National Security and Parliamentary Democracy*, Oxford: Oxford University Press.

McLaughlin, E. (1992) 'The Democratic Deficit: European Union and the Accountability of British Police', *British Journal of Criminology*, Vol. 32, No. 4, 473–87.

Mathias, P. (1995a) 'Justice Seeks Evidence on Mulroney, Moores', *Financial Post*, 18 November, p. 1.

Mathias, P. (1995b) 'Mulroney's Suit Faces Heavy Odds: Experts', *Financial Post*, 21 November, p. 5.

Mathias, P. (1999) 'Swiss Find no Link to Mulroney in Accounts', *National Post*, 3 September, p. 1.

Mawby, R. I. (1990) *Comparative Police Issues*, London: Unwin Hyman.

Nadelman, E. A. (1993) *Cops across Borders: The Internationalization of US Criminal Law Enforcement*, University Park PA: Pennsylvania State University Press.

Palango, P. (1994) *Above the Law: The Crooks, the Politicians, the Mounties, and Rod Stamler*, Toronto: McClelland and Stewart.

La Presse (1995) 'La Suisse enquête sur des pots-de-vin versés à des politiciens canadiens', dimanche, 12 novembre, pp. 1–2.

Sallot, J. (1997) 'Secrecy Hides Airbus Probe', *Globe and Mail*, 8 January, pp. 1 and A4.

Sheptycki, J. W. E. (1996) 'Law Enforcement, Justice and Democracy in the Transnational Arena: Reflections on the War on Drugs', *International Journal of the Sociology of Law*, Vol. 4, No. 1, pp. 61–75.

66   *Jean-Paul Brodeur*

Sheptycki, J. W. E. (1997) 'Faire la police dans la Manche: l'évolution de la co-opération transfrontalière (1968–1996)', *Cultures et Conflits*, Édition Spécial: *Contrôles: Frontières-Identités: Les enjeux autour de l'immigration et de l'asile*, Vols 26/27, Summer-Autumn, pp. 93–123.

Sheptycki, J. W. E. (1998a) 'Policing, Postmodernism and Transnationalisation', *British Journal of Criminology*, Vol. 38, No. 3, 485–503.

Sheptycki, J. W. E. (1998b) 'Police Co-operation in the English Channel Region 1968–1996', *European Journal of Crime, Criminal Law and Criminal Justice*, Vol. 6, No. 3, pp. 216–35.

Sheptycki, J. W. E. (1998c) 'The Global Cops Cometh: Reflections on Transnationalization, Knowledge Work and Policing Subculture' *British Journal of Sociology*, Vol. 49, No. 1, pp. 57–74.

Simpson, Jeffrey (1997) 'The Airbus Affair Concludes with Tough Questions about the RCMP', *Globe and Mail*, 10 January, p. A18.

Der Spiegel (1995) 'Konto mit Code-Wort', No. 14.

3 Liaison officers in Europe

New officers in the European security field

Didier Bigo

Introduction

A new specialist has emerged in policing organisations in Europe, viz: the liaison officer. We might stop to consider why the emergence of this new role should concern us. There are relatively few of them and they are marginal to the central mission of their respective police institutions; but the creation of this specialism is symptomatic of profound changes in our vision of crime and insecurity and of our view of the police agents who seek to control such social disorder. They are also symptomatic of our conceptions about the future of the European Union and of our relations with security (Bigo 1994, 1996). Such transformations are themselves related to practical transformations affecting the different specialised police forces targeting terrorists, drug dealers, or those whose job it is to control illegal immigration (Bigo and Leveau 1992; Benyon et al. 1993; Sheptycki 1995, 1997b). The principles of free trade and free movement have made the liaison officer role crucial for policing in Europe, because it is they who manage the flow of information between their respective agencies. Indeed, police, customs and immigration agencies have all sought to develop specialist liaison officers and the development of various bilateral and multilateral agreements have more or less codified these emergent networks. The resultant interconnection of the various agencies involved (including security agencies; *haute polices*) has served to reinforce the power, status and influence of all.

The legal framework that has emerged on the back of these developments has led to the rise of a new type of specialised government officer, responsible for European matters within the home and justice departments (and more recently within the gendarmerie) (Fijnaut 1991; Monar and Morgan 1995). This takes justice and home affairs matters into the realm of foreign affairs, for example by involving these ministries in negotiating divergent positions and interests relating to immigration. Transnational police concerns with immigration control have extended the reach of these agencies, to the extent that it has even helped determine immigration and asylum policy. In the Franco-Algerian or Germano-Turkish cases, for example, Home Ministries have been important actors in the development and conduct of government policies. What is notable is the siege mentality that has emerged around the issues of immigration and asylum as the topics of religious fundamentalism, terrorism, drugs, delinquency and the image of the immigrant have become somehow fused. This fusion is partly fuelled by the collapse of the bipolar system at the end of the Cold War, which has left the military with no clearly defined enemy. The result has been a perceived common interest between police and military personnel on these questions and this has brought about a decompartmentalisation of the home and defence departments and the constitution of a 'security field'.

This chapter proceeds in two steps. Firstly, some elements concerning the number, the role and the relative importance of the liaison officers and an estimation of the consequent weight of those agencies which are brought together by their mediations will be presented. Secondly, the salient theoretical formulations regarding these shifts in control will be reviewed and a synthesis which aims to reformulate the paradigm that relates to questions about security in Europe will be put forward.

The liaison officer in Europe: professional networks

The importance of liaison officers stationed outside their respective countries cannot be estimated by simple recourse to an estimation of their numbers. There may be no more than a few dozen such officers stationed in any one country, but their role is crucial. It is so because they occupy key posts for the management and exchange of information, they help constitute a web which policy documents and texts emanating from the European Union, the European Council and other institutions – subnational, national and transnational – refer to as 'internal security'. They ensure that data centres, like the Schengen Information System, Supplementary Information Request at the National Entry (SIRENE) and Europol, are new centres of power; new centres for the surveillance of the populations who make the European territory their home.

If we want truly to understand how the Europeanisation of security came about we must step away from a nominalist or essentialist view –

there is nothing natural about the Europeanisation of the problems that have been grouped under the label internal security; it is a political process. The networks themselves are the product of contingency. For example, there are the many bilateral agreements that have grown up to deal with specific problems in the extended zones which demarcate particular border regions. The problems which the various police agencies seek to address in these circumstances are a reflection of the cross-border life of certain regions (Benelux and the North of France; the Spanish and French areas of the Basque country together with Catalonia, are examples here). Such police problems that there are in these regions are restricted to specific zones, there is no 'strategic depth' to this police activity. There is no evidence that there is a strategic interlinking of organised crime groups across and between these regions; no transnational Mafia. The problems presented for the policing of terrorism (Action Direct and the German Red Army Faction) in the 1970s produced a similar recourse to bilateralism (and, in some instances, trilateral ties), in part because the existing European mechanisms were, at the time, considered too large and unwieldy to respond with the necessary speed. Regarding international drugs trafficking the situation has been very different. Historically, the response of police agencies has extended well beyond the European territory (Nadelmann 1993b). The issue of migration seems similar to this latter case. It can be convincingly argued that real 'work of politicisation' has been required in order to make the European arena (that is: the EU) an appropriate institutional setting for dealing with these various forms of criminality. This process is fraught and, despite repeated attempts, there are still no standard criteria for what might constitute 'Eurocrime' (Sheptycki 1995). This does not limit the evident need for a formalisation of the operational frame, including the legal dimension, for policing in Europe. The Schengen agreement remains, perhaps, the best model yet to be actualised in this regard.

  The 1970s is the watershed for this process of Europeanisation of crime and police issues. It was during this period, and partly in response to American attempts to control Interpol, that what might best be described as 'security clubs' (Berne, Quantico, Vienna, Pompidou, Star, etc.) were created. This was accompanied by the creation of TREVI (an intergovernmental framework established by the European Council of Ministers for policing terrorism) during the period (T1, in 1976) and its later expansion (T2, in 1980; T3 in 1985; and, somewhat confusingly, T 1992 in 1988). At the end of this phase came the Schengen implementing convention in 1990, the creation of the third pillar of Maastricht and establishment of the Europol drugs unit, the setting up of UCLAF (Unité pour Coordination de la Lutte Anti-Fraude) and, finally, the signing of the Europol Convention. The factors that propelled these developments were obvious: fears about political violence and radical fundamentalism, tales of urban insecurity, and immigration issues fused with concerns about the so-called 'fourth freedom': the freedom of movement. While images of disorder in civil society created a specific trajectory of development, the manifest rivalry between different branches of the social control apparatus (police, gendarmerie, customs, immigration officials), both within and between the various national structures, set the process off on a wild dynamic. Into this constellation of developments stepped the new agents of the Europeanisation of crime control, the liaison officers. These agents reinforced both their own presence and the various notions of European security in a dynamic discursive presentation of their own interests. This is, in John Benyon's terms, the 'meso level'; an intermediary stratum between the level of the European political élite and the level of operational policing (Benyon 1992). Its creation was one of the most significant aspects of the Europeanisation of crime control. We can describe this agent as a hybrid jurist/police official, more interested to police the politics of the European field than in policing in the more widely understood sense of the term. Their mission is twofold: in the face of resistance from operational agents they will attempt to codify and institutionalise operational policing, in the face of resistance from the higher echelons of the political sphere they will seek to place this under the rule of law which provides a canopy under which the discretionary practices of police agents can be maintained. The basis of the resistance is obvious enough: for the police, they will seek to minimise bureaucratic drag. For the politicians, they will seek to maximise their own room for political manoeuvring via the notion of sovereignty.

Hence, while Europeanisation is a political strategy pursued by some, but not all, European governments aimed at a successful balance of power politics in Europe – and in which the USA plays a significant extra-continental role – it is also a political strategy played by substate actors from the different social control services in order to maximise their own resource base. Their claim is a need to 'modernise' the technical capacities of their services and to homogenise towards the standards of Europe. This mix of forces played out on the broad terrain of Europe has produced an almost unimaginably complex process and the historical outcome of Europeanisation cannot be predicted. The enlargement of the community to include Scandinavia and the Committee of European Economic Cooperation (CEEC) is likely to cause a de-coupling of the arenas dealing with internal security, freedom of movement and the formal arena of the Union. The potential of this for Europol is the question of whether to extend itself to the police officials of the CEEC. However, Schengen might be the best example for the 'laboratory of the Union', since it may come to include countries like Norway and Switzerland, which refused entry to the EU itself (Keohane and Hoffman 1991; Sheptycki 1998c). Thus, the Europeanisation of insecurity cannot be explained by recourse to the Europeanisation of crime. It is not the product of functional spill-over. It lies in the networks of the different agencies and their struggles for mastering the 'nodes' of communication and of power which favour certain governments or services at the expense of others (cf. Sheptytcki 1997a). Of course, the European Union itself is a coalescence of national territories and is not at all homogeneous. Despite this, there is a real political process of Europeanisation which calls for unceasing negotiations which continuously call into question the principles, indeed rhetoric, concerning threats to sovereignty and the need for control within the defined frontiers (Hurwitz and Lequesne 1991; Quermonne 1992).

Each police agency in Europe has its own control culture, in part based on obvious national differences: the carrying of arms, routine identity checks of citizens or of hotel registrations are some examples which come to mind. To members of a specific control culture such powers seem natural. With Europeanisation they are denaturalised, such powers seem arbitrary and inappropriate. Within the broader field of Europe, the specificity and legitimacy of particular control cultures becomes questionable (cf. Bayley 1992; Brodeur 1983; Gleizal et al. 1993; Reiner 1992). This modifies the way police action is viewed and sometimes revives issues which have been long buried since the inception and successful legitimisation of the various national police forces. The discourse on harmonisation sometimes masks these problems but produces other more serious ones. The routine identity check carried out according to the Schengen Convention is motivated by a kind of rationality different from that of the earlier frontier checks concerning foreigners. All those who pass the frontier are now suspected of being potential criminals, especially if they do not look like 'Europeans'; like white and wealthy people. Even the most passing references to these political accords carry with them semantic elements which show significant shifts in how (in)security is being perceived – an illustration of these theoretical questions of both the legitimacy and suitability of these measures may clarify this point.

Analysis of practices

There are many significant questions. What are the rationalities for solidarity between the different national police forces and between the different security agencies? How is a greater sense of identity forged between them? What are the binding motives of these control cultures? How do the affinities and rivalries operate? Through national solidarity? Professional solidarity? What are the shared representations of controllers and how do they make sense of their daily activities? What do they do daily?

This link between a sociology of the practices of small groups and the types of rationality which structure these practices is rarely carried to its end. However, only a detailed account of these social practices – so often ignored in the academic literature or, worse, romanticised in the journalistic accounts – can allow us to move away from the different levels of legitimisation proposed by the actors (or, indeed, all too often by the researchers). Such legitimisation can be observed to operate as claims about explanations of hidden and deeper truths which have to be revealed because they are so deeply buried. Ultimately grand causes, corresponding to grand effects, are evoked, bearing labels such as national police traditions, centralised or decentralised models, or the sovereignty/integration duality (Monjardet 1985). This will not be our approach. It is not necessary to look for grand causes behind these practices. It is these practices and their 'contours' which have to be studied. Paul Veyne (1984, 1990) and Michel Foucault (1977, 1980, 1991) have shown the importance of these practices and the danger of reifying so-called grand causes and of mere incorporation of practices into models or ideologies. Thus, if we are to consider what the actors say in a serious way, if we ask questions about their statements, about what they say in texts (knowledge) but also in their way of carrying out checks of persons, about the logic of surveillance, about the management of data (power) and finally about the conditions in which they move, then our vision begins to change. Because it is in their most ordinary work, that which they do every day (and not in their possible secret missions), that we note tangible marks of crucial transformations which are affecting 'governality' within the European boundaries. It is these practices which help us to understand the link which exists between the habitus of the actors and the field from which they emerge (cf. Bourdieu 1990; Giddens 1990; Luhmann 1995).

Police officers abroad: new transnational agents

Based on interviews carried out with over one hundred police officers (in the main specialist liaison officers responsible for the prevention of terrorism, drugs and organised crime) and members of the criminal justice complex and security forces (gendarmes, judges, customs officers and members of the armed forces) in France and abroad (in declining order of interview contacts: Belgium, the Netherlands, the UK, Ireland, Spain, the USA, French-speaking sub-Saharan Africa, Italy, Germany, Greece, Portugal and Central America) it is possible to make some specific observations. These relate to both specific police working practices and to the particularities of officers who have an interest in Europe, not only due to their origins, but also to their career paths.

These officers are at the margins of the police world, the sphere that they inhabit is altogether different from that of local uniformed officers, detectives, or investigating officers, regardless of rank. These police officers are often multi-lingual and have some form of advanced education, usually including university. Typically, they recognise each other as belonging to the same 'small world', a world which is élitist and political, but one which involves an unsure career trajectory – certainly less sure than colleagues in more traditionally recognised positions in their respective organisations. Some officers, particularly those with investigative experience, regard this unusual career tangent as a means of promotion, but some are parachuted into the European archipelago for a change of scenery after an unsatisfying experience in a previous posting. More often such officers are given such duties after past successful endeavours – in such instances financial and symbolic benefits are evident.

Without systematic study any generalisation is impossible and national differences in recruiting practices also need to be taken into account. On the whole these officers are part of a cohort who consider diplomas, and attendant signifiers of credentialism as valuable, even though such indicators remain subordinate to 'street-level experience' which remains the *sine qua non* of the police world view. They understand themselves to be knowledge workers and argue in favour of a scientific police force, with more desk work, strategic analysis, and analytical skills and correspondingly less emphasis on the 'action cult' (Sheptycki 1998a). This distance makes them somewhat sceptical about public policies for crime control, and their ability to make accurate comparisons between states gives them a sense of proportion. Consequently they do not much resemble the typical caricature: the anti-intellectual, conservative, and all too often racist, police officer. On the contrary, very often liaison officers are quite urbane and cosmopolitan. This does not, however, prevent them from viewing the world in terms of (in)security in which modernisation and the technology of control must be forever on the increase in order that the social body not be submerged in a flow of immigrants and criminality. At this level of generalisation this sketch is not inappropriate to the French gendarmes and their European brethren.[1] On the whole, officers of the gendarmes may feel less estranged from their parent forces, given the usually rapid turnover in any one position and a lower level of participation in the European arena, but there are signs of rapid change. Gendarmes have created their own structures within southern Europe particularly (IHESI 1992, 1993a, 1993b, 1993c). They practise a double tactic of autonomy to preserve the identity they originally felt was being threatened by the Europeanisation process whilst actively participating in any European forum where the police force is present. They have their own liaison officers within each structure and insist on being officially represented at all levels.

Liaison officers – an interface role

As residents in a country not their own, these liaison officers, or liaison civil servants as they are sometimes called, play a key role as the human interface between the various national police forces, establishing and maintaining the flow of data between each force repository. An important distinction between bilateral liaison officers (posted abroad in foreign police agencies) and so-called European liaison officers (posted at Europol Headquarters in the Hague) is worth dwelling on.

Bilateral liaison officers

Many bilateral liaison officers have seen their sphere of action widen outside their initial domain through an extension logic which reorients them from the specific fight against either terrorism or drugs to cover a continuum that now includes immigration. From the perspective of France, it would seem that the field of action has been progressively extended, the chronological sequence being from drugs work to terrorism and finally illegal immigration (cf. Sheptycki 1997a). During the 1960s there was nothing like a liaison agent, except within the Interpol organisation (Anderson 1989). In some instances police officers may have received some training abroad or travelled abroad on specific missions, but they were not actually resident outside their home country. During the 1970s a number of French officers were sent to the USA for the first time, in order to work on the drug war (Nadelmann 1993a). This was in the context of the so-called 'French Connection', under an agreement signed between the US and French governments in the wake of the 1972 UN Single Convention on Narcotic Drugs. Those first few officers stayed on, but apparently their salaries were not drawn from the national police budget, nor were they given precise status. This ambiguity took some time to clear up. Indeed, all through the 1970s there are examples of French agents working abroad and this raised questions, not only about financial arrangements, but also about the legal status of such agents. These questions were also manifest in relation to foreign agents working within France. A series of interservice agreements were made in the 1980s which helped the various services involved in this to establish the propriety of reciprocity (Bigo 1996). While the officers in charge of the fight against drugs laid the foundations for the later work in anti-terrorism, that new basis also meant that the qualities of the agents in question had to shift. In the drugs field, such liaison officers were usually assigned to a taskforce dealing with a specific case and, even though their positions were, strictly speaking, non-operational, it is evident from my interviews that this was not always the case (see also, Nadelmann 1993b). In anti-terrorism work, the agents concerned could not work precisely this way – in this case they functioned more as points of contact, as agents through whom confidential information could be passed without recourse to a paper trail. The range of assignment units for agents partly depended on the particular combination of police agencies and what their anti-terrorist strategy consisted of. Thus in Germany, anti-terrorist activities are centralised under the auspices of the Bundeskriminalamt (BKA) and French officers working there with German officers are sent to Wiesbaden.[2] Foreign liaison officers working in France were assigned to the Unité de la Coordination de la Lutte Anti-Terrorisme (UCLAT) which kept them at arms distance from the Directorate de la Surveillance du Territoire (DST) or the Renseignements Généraux (RG).[3] In Belgium a similar structure was established, integrating members of the Gendarmerie from both countries into a forum which had, hitherto, been a strictly police operation. In the Netherlands, such efforts were concentrated in the new Headquarters of the Divisie Centrale Recherche Informatie (CRI) (which houses the Interpol National Central Bureau), after the reorganisation of the police services there. In the UK, liaison officers were placed in the Special Branch offices (European Liaison Section) at New Scotland Yard, as well as the National Criminal Intelligence Services (NCIS) and the Immigration Office. In Italy, they were assigned to the anti-terrorist and organised crime departments within the Arma dei Carabiniere. In Spain, with the particularity of the Basque problem, French liaison officers were either sent to Madrid or to Vittoria in the Basque country.

There were tensions in how these bilateral arrangements for the reciprocal exchange of liaison officers would be conceived and these were partly played out under the umbrella of the TREVI system. France, Italy, Germany and Spain agreed to the principle of informal liaison, but the Dutch and UK governments wished to confer upon their liaison officers official diplomatic status. Some characterised this as 'Americanisation' (since FBI and other law enforcement officers operating overseas have frequently sought to cover themselves through diplomatic immunity) but the idea was that such liaison officers operated as police 'ambassadors' (Sheptycki 1998a). For France, the result of the divergence of views was a series of bilateral agreements. In the period of most rapid growth these were: 13 October 1986, between France and Italy, which foresaw an exchange of experts in anti-terrorism and organised crime; April 1987, between France and Germany, to exchange anti-terrorism information; 29 May 1987, between France and Spain, on terrorism, organised crime and drugs trafficking; 19 May 1989 between France and the UK, on terrorism, organised crime, drugs trafficking and illegal immigration; and 14 June 1991, between France and Belgium, on terrorism, organised crime and drugs. There are also French liaison officers operating abroad outside Europe. By all accounts there are two officers in the USA (Washington since 1971 and Miami since 1980), two in Thailand (since 1977), two in Pakistan (Islamabad and Karachi), two in Colombia, two in the Caribbean (Antilles and Guyana), one for Trinidad and Tobago and two in Cyprus. Significantly, these liaison officers are assigned to the French embassies rather than local law enforcement offices in order to skirt round the reciprocity rule.[4] Lastly, there have also been the officers operating under the TREVI liaison officers scheme; a significant innovation in its time, since such were conceived of in order to assist all European Community forces and not just those of the home country. There has not been any information which would allow outside observers to estimate with any degree of accuracy the number of such officers.

There is one other area for the exchange of liaison officers and this is the fruit of the Schengen agreement which allows for the exchange of such agents in order to control problems related to immigration. In

August 1990 a French liaison officer was sent to Wiesbaden and a German officer was sent to Paris in order to begin the process of analysis of the implications of German reunification and the problems linked to the movement of the external border of the EU to the Oder–Neisse line. In 1993 this was bolstered when a French officer was sent to the Oder–Neisse border and a German officer was sent to the PAF headquarters in Paris. In the wake of the Schengen agreement there has been a flurry of activity and joint police stations have been set up on the Schengen internal (Franco-German and Franco-Spanish) borders in which officers of the respective countries work alongside each other in the same building.[5]

According to my interviews, France has sent 19 bilateral liaison officers to six other European forces and is preparing to add to this number considerably in order to cover all 15 countries as well as to increase the number of officers per country. As of 1998, France had received 11 foreign officers: three Germans, three Spaniards, two Italians, one Briton, one Dutchman, one Belgian. Germany is also quite active with some 25 such officers abroad (four in Spain, two in Portugal, two in France, two in Italy, two in the Netherlands, one in the United Kingdom and others in Turkey, Brazil, Argentina, Thailand) as well as playing host to 15 guest officers. Other countries in Europe have developed, *mutatis mutandis*, along similar lines. It should be pointed out that this causes difficulties for smaller countries; as one official pointed out to me in Luxembourg, if they were to develop their system to this degree, there would be more foreigners in some of their police units than there are Luxembourgeois!

European liaison officers

Officers detailed to Europol Headquarters in the Hague are a new departure from the trend outlined above. Their relationship to their home countries has changed subtly, not that they cease to report and liaise with their home countries, quite the opposite. They continue to be quite dependent on their respective national administrations, but the hundred plus officers that have been dedicated to Europol by the 15 participating countries function as part of a mini-police of Europe and they play a crucial role in the transformations of (in)security at the European level because they are strategically essential to the new methods of control and surveillance of European suspect populations. One of my interviewees likened himself to a 'human contact exchange'. Another added: 'We are like station masters. It is up to us to find the right shunting and direct information as quickly as possible to the place where it is of most use rather than sending it to a marshalling yard, like Interpol, where it is stocked and never used.' Another officer summed up the *modus operandi* in its entirety:

> We put people in contact with one another, overcoming cultural and procedural differences and language problems. We are privileged intermediaries between our home and host countries. And that works in both directions. Of course a lot of our time is spent informing our own services about who is doing what and where in our posting country, but the opposite is also true. People come to see us as soon as they have to contact someone from our side. The term liaison is well chosen. With just a handful of people on either side two police forces are linked together. But this is always entirely voluntary and there is no obligation to go through us.
>
> (from interview)

Other officers spoke to me quite frankly about how the simple fact of working under one roof has transformed the liaison job beyond that of the bilateral arrangements already described.

> We go beyond bilateral exchanges because all the foreign liaison officers present in the host country work in the same building and get to know one another. That allows a very European mentality to develop which goes beyond bilateral relations. This may be less true for our colleagues who are assigned to a particular service in which they are the only foreigner. Here we already make up a miniature Europe. Once Europol is in its place . . . the national units of each country will have a centre, a base, a converging point.

This officer also pointed out that the multitude of different police-type administrations brought together for Euro-policing created such complicated arrangements that '100 per cent of our time is taken up with liaison work . . . we scarcely have time to take part in investigations, particularly because we have no operational authority'. Others acknowledge that there was an inevitable degree of involvement in actual investigations: 'we cannot help ourselves in certain cases from thinking about the investigation at hand and putting the right people in contact with one another . . . we do get involved. On the other hand, we never act alone behind our colleagues' backs as the Americans sometimes do.' This officer stressed the relations of trust that have been built up within the 'small world' of liaison police and decried the development of bureaucratic and legal rules 'which get in the way of our work' characterising them as 'the tragedy of the last twenty years'. The increase in the number of police dedicated to this mission was seen by this officer to be a boon, 'but [there are] not yet enough of us compared to international crime. Only a federal European police force would be able to sort out that problem. We are the precursors.'

Not everyone shares this point of view, nor is every officer in this apparatus enamoured of the federalist project. Some stress that working together through an intergovernmental framework is, first and foremost, a method of increasing efficiency and effectiveness in the fight against European organised crime. Quite simply, some officers remain national police officers abroad. Regardless of personal views on this issue, and many interviewees stressed that this was a personal matter, all seemed to agree the importance of remaining aloof from operational policing and 'sticking to the letter'. Another officer put it this way:

> We are sales representatives, selling the image of our police force abroad. I am not convinced that we are moving towards a 'Holy Alliance' and a federal police force. Too many things keep us apart, maybe it's because I come from the prevention of terrorism. What's sure is that we are often in competition with one another. It's the one who has the best address book, the best network . . . we're also competing to sell our police model outside Europe. You can make a packet that way. Criminal investigation police officers are often less aware of national interests than we are. They have been working together for a long time and have learned from Interpol, but when it comes to terrorism, as for immigration and even drugs, it's a lot less straightforward. In fact that's why we have been created.

As for access to sensitive data, many officers admit that even though they do not have direct access, the bonds of camaraderie mean that they can get hold of the information they are looking for. All insist on the operational applicability of intelligence and the speed of information transmission as the key to modern policing at every level. What we have described here is an original new creation which has changed police practices in Europe by interconnecting the forces and also by interconnecting various fields of activity, all of which had formerly been independent. The liaison officer is the crucial development here. Since widespread interconnection of police files is forbidden, and even undesirable for operational reasons, they have become the human interface for data interconnection (Bigo 1992; Sheptycki 1995).

Other security agents affected by transnationalisation

European legal experts: a new staff

Apart from the liaison officers themselves, police collaboration fosters the development of other transnational specialists, particularly those officials from Interior and/or Justice departments with legal backgrounds. In France, for example, general inspectors who specialise in European affairs establish the framework for political and legal collaboration on internal security. These officials will have the task of institutionalising and legitimising police co-operation at the European level. As one official put it to me, they seek to create 'a formal framework which will enable us to weave a web of rights and obligations that, as far as possible, will cover all the areas of activity of those police officers sent abroad and all the cases of exchange of data or men between national police forces'. This is not an easy task, as another official put it. 'We have to reconcile the irreconcilable, the sovereignty that the Ministers are so attached to with the European integration that certain heads of government are after; the legal protection and codification of activities which allows us to control police officers with the loose rein of informal relations that they want at grass roots.' Further, 'if we want to face the increase in criminality, illegal immigration and terrorism, we have to do all that as quickly as possible and if certain members lag behind we have to leave them by the wayside for the good of a more restricted group that can advance more rapidly, as is the case with Schengen.' This can lead to complaints: 'They want us to do everything at once. To allow free movement within Europe and yet tighten border checks to control migration flows; to maintain an expansive asylum policy and strangle immigration fraud and false documents; to increase collaboration and maintain the prerogatives of sovereignty.' It is worth stressing that the centrality of the doctrine of state sovereignty and the great emphasis on territorial considerations emanate from the lawyers rather than the police officers themselves.

Customs officers: crime and borders

Customs officers know very well that the borders are shifting and changing as a result of the processes of transnationalisation. They see this as a dangerous process. On the one hand, as an institution, customs are threatened by the very notion of free movement of people and goods and have made a collective response as a result. Thus, we can see a certain instrumentality to pronouncements about the ever-increasing flow of illegal goods, drugs, counterfeit products, etc. In response to this, the UK remained adamant about maintaining her border controls. In France there was an initial movement in a similar direction, which was reversed only after introduction of compensatory powers given to customs officials. Customs officers have obtained criminal investigation police powers and can take part in drug-delivery surveillance operations. Customs officers now play a major role all over Europe, linking the issues of crime prevention and immigration as well as the debate on security deficiency and compensatory measures. In joining with the police and gendarmes they have changed the economics of security activity. They have both facilitated security extension at the transnational level and helped to focus it on the frontiers. They have brought whole battalions of men and women with them who, along with the border police (another security force profoundly affected by the notion of free movement), have transformed the Europeanisation of (in)security into one of the determining battlefields not only in the struggle between nations for European domination but also in the conflicts between services at the national level.

Judges: a late but fundamental inclusion

To their amazement and at their expense, judges only discovered the extent of the informal police networks within Europe at the signing of Maastricht and only began to adapt their behaviour in the wake of that realisation. Their attempt to 'make up for lost time' brings the examining magistrates into transnational control activities that take them outside their traditionally bounded national territory. Belatedly, networks of judicial officials began to form and, indeed, in some areas by the end of the 1990s, had developed set routines for their activities. However, the diversity of penal codes and the differences in type of procedure (accusatorial or inquisitorial) limit the extent of harmonisation (Harding et al. 1995; Joubert and Bevers 1996). It appears that examining magistrates (in those countries where they exist) are more affected than other types of judges. These magistrates generally feel isolated, misunderstood and out-of-tune with the lawyers working in the various departments of the interior. Nevertheless, their participation is essential in order to legitimise the security measures that are being developed. It is no surprise that, despite their marginal role, all the official headings within the agreements put police and judicial collaboration on an equal footing.

Diplomats and members of parliament: a loss of power?

With reference to issues like drug use and immigration, there is no doubt that civil servants working in 'social ministries' (in the main, health and employment ministries) have seen their role displaced, *vis-à-vis* 'security ministries' (that is: justice and interior ministries). In France the practice of inter-ministerial delegation at prime-ministerial level has limited this loss of influence, but even there the trend is unmistakable. The foreign affairs ministries in most European countries (in some this would be the ministry of European affairs) have also experienced 'turf wars' with civil servants from justice and interior ministries. They have had to endorse decisions that are inimical to their view of the issues at hand and, hence, feel isolated and without a voice. Diplomats who took a hand in the drafting of agreements by which they are now bound, or who have been posted to countries where immigration and asylum are sensitive issues, have difficulty in accepting a downgrading of their status in relation to those domestic ministers who have taken on new roles in international affairs. They seek to regain their position by a twofold strategy. First, new technology for the delivery and control of visas in consular officers is thought to provide a good tool to enhance not only the practice of their work, but the status of their occupation. Second, they also hope that the third pillar of Maastricht will prevent an increase in informal networks among the controllers and give consular officials more control over police activities. In all of this they are counting on the support of elected MPs who sometimes voice similar concerns. Indeed, MPs, be they European or national ones, have criticised the way in which the agreements were drafted and the secrecy that surrounded them. For both Schengen and Europol they, like the diplomats, felt that they were being kept at even more of a distance than usual by the civil servants of the ministries in question. However, they do admit that as they have no authority to amend intergovernmental agreements the only strategy left to them was an all-or-nothing one which forced them to ratify the agreements (Sivanandan 1993).

The armed forces: fusing internal and external security issues?

Since the preoccupation of internal security agencies merges into the international sphere and creates a link between home and foreign affairs, it is not surprising that they come up against military interests. This is particularly the case since the end of the bi-polar world of the Cold War because the military now have an excess of resources in relation to the means at their disposal. In response to a police movement towards transnationalisation, the armed forces are moving in the opposite direction, returning to internal affairs and border protection in search of infiltrated enemies. Thus, concerns over (in)security, not least those entwined with the migration issue, represent a fusing of the security apparatus from the civilian police, to the customs officers and on to the armed forces.

The end of the Cold War has profoundly altered the surface on which the military apparatus rests (Waltz 1993). No longer confined to conflicts which are at the borders of nation-states, they have been accommodated in a newly emerging (in)security apparatus. The new enemies in question are not particularly powerful – the problem does not lie in the economics of power, it lies in the ability to locate the enemy who cannot be immediately identified. Since the new enemy is within the body of society, there is a need for a new strategic military line; no longer so concerned with interstate conflict, the military has a new set of jobs: anti-guerrilla tactics, prevention of terrorism, drugs prohibition enforcement, and international peace-enforcement are just some of them (Clutterbuck 1990; Singer and Wildavsky 1993; Gregory 1996; Brodeur 1997). In all of this there has been an intertwining of military and police technology (Haggerty and Ericson 1999); the armed forces have assumed more responsibility for the maintenance of surveillance of suspect populations (Sheptycki 1998b).

The former separation of internal and external security has been disturbed. Changes in the international context in the recent past have replaced the image of One Big Enemy, with a multitude of unforseeable internal dangers and the very notion of (in)security has been widened to take account of this. This, it is sometimes held, is the product of media manipulation and/or of an American plot to disguise their hegemony. However, if (in)security is coming into the realm of military strategy, and if this strategy is growing in importance, it is neither because of an actual increase in sources of disorder, nor because public opinion demands it, nor is it a result of a plot by the 'big boys'. Rather it is because of the discourse employed by social controllers and other experts in the application of coercive power on behalf of the state which impinges on our lives every day, making them appear less secure through the amplification of perceived 'threats' (see also Sheptycki 1996). The interlocking of internal and external security is not a reflection of an increase in the threats facing modern society. Rather it is a lowering of the threshold of threat acceptance maintained by social controllers in tandem with the upsurge in the use of police methods themselves. The consequent vision produced by security professionals is of a world seemingly less secure. In this respect there is a double movement: in theory the same security programme, with the same coercive solutions and the militarisation of society's preserve, can be applied to both Russian aggression and to anti-social behaviour in children. Even while it is being argued that terrorism, organised crime and the Mafia are on the rise, which demands a reply from the armed forces, police are moving into military domains. Internal solutions are exported to external contexts more often than the reverse. Thus, in Bosnia, soldiers carry out international police operations and ask the gendarmes how to go about keeping the peace without 'degenerating into war'. Meanwhile, inner-city skirmishes have become the training ground for international crises and the methods used in both domains are discussed at the European level as 'proactive policing techniques'. In order to understand these transformations in control and surveillance we have to view them as agents in one and the same field, a field where internal and external (in)security have merged (for a suggestive historical view see: Bayley 1975; Tilley 1985).

Police archipelagos

Thus police officers and others who embody similar control cultures have come to broaden their horizons to include Europe and beyond. Policing is moving away from the local neighbourhood to play a much bigger role on the transnational stage. The old notions based on locale, the social or simply national political considerations, or ones based on a cleavage between state military interests and state police interests, simply no longer make sense. Of course there are still local police stations doing local police work. However, as the spectres of drugs, organised crime, illegal immigration and terrorism (the new horsemen of the apocalypse) loom ever larger, specialist police are becoming more numerous. A large amount of police work now concerns patrolling the data in order to spot connections between criminals, and much of this goes beyond the merely local or even national. Intelligence-led policing transcends the internal/external divide and police officers are increasingly dealing with areas that previously belonged to external intelligence and the army. These developments have not come about without some institutional friction. It is not a seamless conspiratorial web and adaptation to the new modes has been difficult. We might say that the result of this is that co-operation has been better achieved between identical services across different national traditions than it has across services nested within national traditions. This has created police archipelagos that are far less dependent on the requirements of national sovereignty and has facilitated the setting up of networks of control agents who see as their primary task the maintenance of public order, broadly conceived, and who distance themselves from all political reasoning. All over Europe there are thousands of control agents working together every day; in so doing they are breaking down the myth of national sovereignty.

Bridging the disciplines and the hypothesis of a security field

One of the most significant barriers to a concerted analysis of this new security field is undoubtedly the current divisions in disciplinary knowledge that constitute the social sciences. The mere fact of describing the work of police liaison officers is corrosive of the traditional categories of understanding. Thus, one finds oneself on the border of two disciplines which, like parallel lines, are destined never to meet. In disciplinary terms those are: sociology (of policing) and international relations.

Of course the sociology of policing has a number of good studies to its credit which have created solid links between sociology, criminology, history and law. And the sociology of the military has sought to emulate this, perhaps with less success. The solid Anglo-Saxon tradition of police sociology has been joined by some new French studies (Guyomarch 1991; Journés 1993; Monjardet and Lévy 1995; Bigo 1996). A political science of control cultures has developed. This political science of policing had already begun to ponder the changes in the national police forces from the moment they began to co-operate beyond national frontiers in the European framework and thought about co-ordinating their efforts in various organisations (e.g. Interpol, TREVI, Europol). It tended to describe the police forces of the different countries separately. It busied itself with large battalions of the police institutions, with the constraints of the profession, with the police officers' unions. But the political science of policing considered the small groups of government officials posted abroad as marginal. Its practitioners became interested in the game of comparing the similarities and differences of police forces within the European Union, asking abstract questions about their compatibility and the outline of the best possible models for police organisation, but they have scarcely begun to analyse the dynamics of interdependence, the effects of transnationalisation, the processes of Europeanisation – excepting, perhaps for a few pioneering studies (Anderson 1989; Anderson et al. 1995). This has begun to change. As Nadelmann (1993a and b) has pointed out with reference to Drug Enforcement Agency (DEA) and Federal Bureau of Investigation (FBI) officials, who are operating outside US jurisdiction in increasing numbers, we need to cross the usual intellectual boundaries in order to propose working hypotheses which draw upon international relations as well as criminology. While the study of international relations has sometimes stressed the need to examine internal relations between different bureaucratic entities within states, this discipline does not, by and large, concern itself with the internal politics of states, this largely because of the dominance of 'neo-realism' (Keohane and Nye 1970; Keohane 1989). Thus, scholars of international relations have historically not taken an interest in the international games played by police agencies, except for some attention paid to terrorism and drug control. The idea of studying these people – who worked outside their national territory but who, nevertheless, clearly belonged to bureaucracies nominally geared towards internal matters – never occurred to the proponents of the neo-realist approach. They were worried about finding the seeds of transnationalism in the very heart of the state, that is among state actors operating at levels below that of the designated national representatives (diplomats, foreign envoys and the like). Similarly, military sociology in France confined itself to the study of the personnel and severed all links with strategy, as if these were questions for two radically distinct disciplines. The idea that the sociology of military personnel and discussions of strategic questions could be mutually informative has been consistently waved aside. The renewal of the transnationalist school has undoubtedly shown the artificiality of these boundaries.

Ethan Nadelmann is one of the first people to grasp the significance of this transgression of disciplinary boundaries, and his explanation does not depend on suggestions that transnational crime has grown and thus requires a transnational police response. Rather, he has shown that it is the redefinition of certain (long-standing) activities as criminal. However, because of his (admittedly important) focus on the internationalisation of American law enforcement, he misses the connections to the issue of migration and, further, to the fusion of internal and external security. Peter Katzenstein is also well aware of the dangers of the segmentation of knowledge and he has sought to analyse the problems of internal and external security as a whole (see for example: Katzenstein 1990, 1996), although he juxtaposes them without fully restructuring these ideas. Nevertheless, he was among the first to point out that the end of bi-polarity meant that the military and other security services would turn to more diffuse threats (terrorism, organised crime), phenomena already dealt with by police-type agencies, as a way of maintaining their institutional necessity. It was the boundary between the field of knowledge which had to be pulled down so that a new coherent field of analysis could emerge. This new field crosses the line usually traced by the social sciences between the external and the internal, between defence and police problems, between problems of national security and problems of public law and order. It brings into its purview military and police forces and all the other professionals of threat management.

The notion of a security field and a critique of traditional approaches to international policing

The notion of a 'security field' is largely inspired by Pierre Bourdieu. He understands a field to be a network or configuration of objective relations between positions. Such positions are defined objectively in their existence and in the determinations which they impose on their occupants, agents or institutions, whose present and potential situation in the structure of distribution of different kinds of powers (or of capital) yields access to the specific profits which are at stake in the field and result from their objective relations to the other positions (Bourdieu 1990). But the bureaucratic milieu under study here does not have different types of capital (economic, cultural or symbolic) which would permit us to differentiate the positions. Rather we have a distribution of positions depending on types of knowledge (for threat management) which permit types of statement (in Foucault's meaning of the term) which each agency is trying to promote. It should be evident that our approach here is a fusion or crossed reading of Bourdieu and Foucault rather than an application of a single grid of meaning. Such an approach shows the evident limitations of either a functionalist interpretation or an anti-civil-liberties thesis, which are the most common explanations for the phenomenon under study: police co-operation.

The functionalist vision of police co-operation

A certain functional teleology is evident from a reading of the knowledge that is produced by the European Commission and the European Parliament. This holds that police institution building follows in the wake of the processes of European supra-state construction on the one hand and trans-European crime networks on the other. Historical inevitability on its side, it is hardly worth pursuing the study of the internal political struggles, as the various occupational cultures of the various nation-state agencies battle for dominance in order eventually to define the administrative remit of the new Europolice. A political opposition to this teleology stems from a desire to restate the principles and values of the nation-state, this is expressed in juridical terms in the French context. It is in this domain that the notion of sovereignty conflicts with the functional logic of federalism. This explains the de-linking of an intergovernmental Europe (the Schengen Convention) and a European Community as well as the twists and turns along the catwalk of the third pillar of Maastricht (Art. 100, Art. K9). All could be explained as the dialectical opposition of sovereignty and federalism played out on the juridical field. In this picture we see Germany as the federalist, Britain as the sovereigntist and France occupying the golden mean, thus allowing the building of Europe without betraying sovereignty. Not everyone shares the point of view of the French *énarches*. To this mix could be added the notions of separate national police cultures, or styles, which might operate as a drag on institution building. In this view, sovereignty is a Franco-British ideology, not so much a fundamental principle of the state, but the legitimisation of a certain idea of the state. The real difficulties lie elsewhere. The many and various police forces are the product of specific national histories which have yielded different police–society relations (Sheptycki 1999). Certain countries have known the police controlled by central authorities, others have known only local police controlled closely by the local population. This discourse is more subtle, but has a tendency to perceive the various national cultures as homogeneous and antagonistic entities. It is interesting to note that many players in social control apparatus share similar views. Pluralism is one of the sub-variants in the functionalist debate. This notion of a Europe of nation-states is infused with the theme of economic globalisation and the inescapable development of a neo-federal state. Here the national cultures have spontaneously given birth to different national police models which clash and slow the homogenisation of Europe. This process, however, is as irresistible as glaciation, as the various nation-states are gradually metamorphosed into a larger state as part of a civilisation trend towards a post-Weberian state. This state is less coercive, more co-operative, a state turned more to economy than security. In this view the cultural variable explains the political game, but the global trend remains obscure.

The second tangent of functionalism is also frequently expressed. This holds that the Europeanisation of police force is explained by the Europeanisation of crime. This is the province of the official report: Euro-terrorism, drug trafficking, trans-border crime, fraud against the European Union, all can be brought forward as justifications for a police agency evolved to the task. Almost all official reports reiterate through statistical indicators the idea that crimes and threats are increasing, especially on the frontiers of Europe, and this justifies the need to strengthen police collaboration. Any number of academic studies do much the same; after presenting statistical facts and figures they ponder over the possible adaptations of police and, if they are more critical about the statistical models and more doubtful about the political stakes, they still do not think about the meaning of this relation of functional adaptation. It is not my intention to suggest that changes in crime have had no effect on the police organisation, simply to say that there is no linear causality between the two and to suggest that the actors of security always interpret these changes in a specific manner (Marx 1981). We can say, with Mary McIntosh (1975), that the world of crime and the world of police are semi-autonomous. The police world cannot be interpreted in the simple terms of 'reactivity' to a given stimulus of violence. In other words, even if relations characterised as rivalry or 'technical competition' exist between the *underworld* and the *upperworld*, the latter is not solely determined by changes in the forms of deviance which, in any case, is always *officially* designated. The police world is, in part, the creator of its own norms which derive from internal processes and institutional stakes. Police interpret the underworld according to their own construction of the threat; it is their interpretation that gives it a specific meaning (Berger and Luckmann 1967). This suggests that there is a complex and dialectical relation between the already embedded police tendency to label and the forms of acts potentially labelled as criminal. There is a correlation between the evolution of certain forms of crime, which are made significant at a given time and in a given set of political circumstances, and the structures of social control that exist. We thus see not an adaptation to an objective reality, but rather a process of perception and definition carried out by parties interested to delineate problems for which they already have the solutions. Only some phenomena amenable to categorisation as crime are defined as such by politicians and policy-makers: terrorism, drug trafficking, organised crime (what could that mean?), and immigration. Problems such as road safety or environmental degradation are left out of this discourse of police co-operation. A political economy of crime labels is evident, since it is clear that those who lay claim to budgetary resources within the dominant terms of crime control discourse will have an advantage over those who use alternative terminology. To use the terms of functional adaptation to explain, without reference to the principles of struggle over the terms of (control) discourse, renders this form of analysis of little utility. Such an approach shows an historical *naïveté*, it is nothing

more than the importation of the preoccupations of the political world
into the construction of the object (crime) rather than a science of the
politics of crime and the cultures of control (Lacroix 1985).

Police co-operation as police conspiracy

The concept of 'field' also allows us to show that there is no cabal – be
it based within a faction of politicians, or of police officials, or both –
conspiring to undermine civil liberties and increase the powers of
police agencies. Rather, a field has emerged which is the result of the
ongoing struggles between actors. Having said this, we can identify
two variants of the conspiracy thesis. The stronger of the two plays on
the theme of postindustrial capitalism, it is a clarion call to the labour
movement intended to rally the proletariat to resist the transnational
bureaucracy of the police (one example of this is Chomsky 1991, especially pp. 108–35). The weaker version makes a distinction between
the 'trustworthy' police professional, who is merely trying to fulfil
legitimate institutional aims, and the deceptions of those who are attempting to manipulate crime discourse in order to boost the career
trajectories of mini-Machiavellis. This instrumental distinction reduces
the scope of the conspiracy, but does not challenge its existence. We
would argue that control talk emerges within a context of bureaucratic
struggles over fiscal resources engaged in by actors who occupy different positions within the same security field. Far from being an alliance
of bullies against the weaklings, the truth régime of social control is
the product of intense struggles concerning the objectives, technical
means and *modus operandi* of the controllers themselves. Indeed, so
intense is the struggle between the various factions within the control
culture (say, between the architects of Europol and the 'new' – post-
1986 – Interpol) that it can potentially cloud our perception of the fact
that the controllers have, by and large, the same interests and the same
feel for the game. The irony is that it is through this struggle against
each other that the overall authority of the control culture is upheld
and this persuades us that the solutions to the problems of (in)security
are in the hands of the controllers and them alone.

  In this connection, it is important to stress that the crime/immigra-
tion linkage is not the simple imagining of conservative politicians and
police agents. It cannot be reduced to the age-old rhetorical game of
the scapegoat (Tannenbaum 1938). It is not a pure 'story' of the élites
which is merely endorsed by the professionals of security. Rather, a
linkage between the broader social world and the special discourse of
the controllers is both evident and necessary to sustain these specialist

truth claims. The régime of truth concerning the crime/immigration nexus is the product of the knowledge work done by police, judicial officials, social scientists and 'mediacrats'. Such knowledge is not simply 'untrue', baseless ideology, it is knowledge that has some foundation. It is necessary to point this out because some authors, inspired by postmodernist relativistic reasoning, have the tendency to forget ontology altogether. In this vein of writing, the deconstruction of security discourses becomes the sole end of the intellectual's labour, the alpha and omega of analysis. Perhaps there is something fundamental in their reasoning, but it is but a small step in the analysis. One has to understand the production of police knowledge and the way in which its manufacture is part of broader truth conditions. It is only in this way that we can hope to understand how this type of knowledge can hold such credence beyond the specialised domain of the controllers. One has to understand the vagaries of power and knowledge within the security field and how this gives rise to its own credibility and thus ensures the spread of this knowledge beyond the confines of the control culture. The concept of the security field is a necessary means to this end.

The concept of the security field

The concept of the security field helps us to understand the dynamics of change occurring within police and military institutions in Europe. Such a conceptual device allows us to transcend the conceptual dichotomies of internal/external and national/international. The parameters of this social space are defined by the different positions of a whole variety of control agencies operating in Europe. The list of such agencies is impressive; we include not only the forces of the regular police and gendarmes, but also border police, immigration and customs officials, the military and security services. We must keep in mind that each of these agencies is embedded within a tradition peculiar to its nation-state (so we have the centralisation of the French police, the federalisation of the German, the territorial and functional decentralisation of the UK police, etc.). It also includes extra-European controllers, of which the DEA and the FBI are prime examples. The field is defined by the place that the various agencies occupy within their respective national political frameworks as well as within the transnational networks of which they are a part. Although it is, at least in part, conditioned by the political struggles that constitute the process of Europeanisation, it is not subordinate to it. Indeed, since the participating agencies are perpetually scouting for cross-border alliances, the evolution of the security field anticipates the evolution of the broader political arena. We can see this clearly in the examples of ties between Europol and the CEEC, or in the developing relations between the Schengen countries and the Nordic Union and Switzerland, or tangentially, in relations between the Eurocorps and NATO.

Thus, the social space operates as a field of forces whose very necessity is ultimately asserted by those who are involved in the competition to define its interests. That these various actors achieve a certain homogeneity of action is a product of similar definitions of the 'adversary'. If the immigrant is the archetypal outsider, it is because of a convergence of various attributes of insecurity attached to him – associations with drugs, petty crime, political subversion by the police and security forces and, more broadly, with high unemployment statistics, or high birth rates and even miscegenation within the general population. In this discursive field, integration ideology is an important component of insecuritisation, since integration is perceived as beneficial not on the grounds of social development and the benefits of cosmopolitanism, but because it is a guard against future revolts. This is a significant feature of (in)security discourse; by globalising terms, fusing phenomenal elements and eliding differences of meaning it facilitates the passage from one reference object to another and enhances the focus effect. For the intellectual, this permeability of terminology is not accounted for by reference to a simple change of perception, it has its origins in the practices and the advancement of technical know-how. If we want to analyse the changes in knowledge, we have to link such changes to observed practices rather than to secondary rationalisations which the actors use to describe their way of doing things. In this instance observations of routine activity and/or the impact of improved technologies become more important than the representations, perceptions and discourses provided by the actors about their respective roles. In order to understand the 'stance' of a particular actor we have to analyse it in relation to the actor's position within the field of security professionals. The stereotypes portrayed by police agents stem from the economics of struggle going on within the field. The end result is the construction of social reality, specifically that which is supposed to threaten us, by specific agents within a given field. This analysis shares an affinity with that of Donatela Della Porta (1995), insofar as she also tries to understand the social construction of reality and the role that police knowledge(s) play in specific forms of life. In her, and our, conception, police knowledge(s) do not consist of neutral terms, they are 'devices of visibility', they are a codified expression of struggles between professionals of the security field and agents of other social fields. A picture of reality (world disorder) is built up through a process of collage which gives pride of place to specific pieces of imagery (immigrant drug dealers and ethnic crime gangs) even while obscuring other images (immigrants as victims of crime). In the end we are left with a distorted *bricolage* masquerading as realism. Thus, even if we have our facts correct about the numbers of immigrants and the numbers of crimes they are involved in, this is not the explanation as to why the immigrant–crime link seems so salient. This makes real sense when we acknowledge the part that is played by our presuppositions about the stranger as a potential criminal and the absolute belief in the necessity of anticipating the negative effects of international disorder surrounding Europe on every side. This is the basis of a moral panic where the immigrant is the folk devil who most threatens our social tranquillity, a pathetic image when we consider that it is the might of the Soviet military machine that this bedraggled army is supposed to replace in the firmament of our fear.

We can thus see that the field is not defined by the power of coercive force, as Weber or Hobbes suggest, but rather by the capacity to produce images of the other who is to be controlled and the consequent polarisation between 'us and them'. This is important, because minor shifts in our way of seeing the picture put before us create a different play of light and shadow. Certain illegalities which were once a matter of priority, slip from the frame and others which were once a matter for tolerance, become highlighted. A new picture of criminality, one which juxtaposes the criminal and the immigrant so closely that they become two halves of the same image, comes into view. In the field of (in)security everything happens as if linked by a continuum of threats which binds terrorism, drugs, organised crime, smugglers, illegal immigrants and asylum-seekers into an apocalyptic vision. The 'security continuum' which emerges from these connections is one of threats arbitrarily defined and unified in a global discourse of disorder. All of the elements of this continuum are the products of police knowledge systems, but we are not obliged to accept all knowledge which purports to describe the facts of our (in)security, even if it is the product of those who claim an authoritative monopoly of such knowledge. Indeed, we should be sceptical, since such knowledge comes precisely from the very people whose habitus is structured by the systematic search for the capacity to manage any threat or risk. The intellectual might do better to contest the diffusion of the truth which has been produced by the myopia of the security field, countering with other social constructions which provide an alternative means to conceive and address the so-called threats identified through the (in)security discourse of the security field.

Conclusion: the providers of security – new forms of governality and the post-Hobbesian state

This chapter has surveyed the many providers of (in)security in the context of the emerging transnational state system in Europe. We need not rearticulate this diverse institutional array which so preoccupies us, suffice to say that it extends from the most mundane municipal police agency to the higher reaches of the intelligence services and the military. These actors in the security field, despite their diversity, can be defined as professionals of threat management, they are producers of a knowledge-power based on (in)security. The main source of their power is not in their capacity to muster coercive force (although they can certainly do that), rather it is in their capacity to define the sources of our insecurity and to produce techniques to manage them. It is too early to tell what the outcome of the consummation of the domains of internal and external security will be. There are both centripetal and centrifugal forces at work. It is not inconceivable that a temporary revival of the military threat from Russia could reintroduce a cleavage which would bring back an earlier police/military division of labour. On the other hand, the continuance of 'peace enforcement' and other humanitarian missions outside Europe looks rather likely. If the latter trend holds, we would be moving towards new forms of governality, which are noticeably more transnational, and in which the role of coercive force would be rather different from that depicted by traditional political science theory.

Neil Walker (1994) has explored one line of research which suggests that the evolution of police co-operation in Europe is symptomatic of broader processes of state transformation. In this transformation, the state, as traditional monopoly holder of the capacity to use force in order to maintain social order within a limited territory, gives way to a post-Hobbesian vision that is transnational (see also Streeck and Schmitter 1991). In discussing the relation between frontiers and population flows, Malcolm Anderson (1996) has addressed the factors which push governments to establish border controls as important symbols of state control. This raises questions about the effective existence of the monopoly of coercion within the territory on the one hand, and the extent to which the state use of force is confined within internationally recognised borders, on the other. If globalisation reduces the power of states within their territory – if, that is, the locus of authority is no longer territorial – frontiers may come to have no meaning. The territorial state may cease to be the fundamental form of governality and the logic of domination will freely cross national boundaries in order to develop a new disciplinary focus on networks. Control bureaucracies might then be freed from the juridical limits set by frontiers. This would also increase the scope for private actors (private security companies, the 'in-house' security providers for multinational companies, or, less comforting, Mafia-type organisations) to play a role in transnational social control. Remote control policies, whereby agents of social control attempt to maintain the security of Western populations by establishing checkpoints and control stations in defined zones of disorder far away from their home territory, might become the norm. The transnationalisation of control bureaucracies, whose operating range has been opened up by the new communications technologies and whose capacity for managing suspect populations has been greatly enhanced by the development of computers, is already happening. The bureaucracies of security that have grown up in the Western states might well redefine themselves, further increasing their capacity for concerted action outside the Western sphere, particularly insofar as those far-flung populations may become mobile and seek to emigrate to greener pastures or engage in forms of prohibited trade. Such a picture is neither predictive of a bypassing of the state, leaving it powerless, nor is it predictive of maximal global security. Rather, it is a confirmation of a form of securisation which Foucault (1989) already anticipated, namely the evolution of the territory-based state to one based on population and the transformation of the modalities of governality, producing a hybrid of the territorial and the ethnic, the coercive and the proactive, together with technological sophistication and the age-old disciplines of the body.

Notes

1 I am thinking here of the Belgian Gendarmerie, the Maréchaussée of Luxembourg and the Netherlands, the Spanish Guardia Civil, The Italian Carabinieri and the Garda Finanza as well as the Austrian Gendarmerie and the German Bundesgrenschutz, all of which bear a genealogical relation to the French Gendarmerie.
2 The BKA is the Federal Criminal Investigations Department. It is the centre for co-operation between the federal and state law enforcement agencies in Germany. Its Headquarters are in Wiesbaden which also houses the Interpol NCB. Anti-terrorist activities are co-ordinated within this organisation under the Koordinierungsgruppe Terrorismusbekämpfung (KGT).
3 The DST is the French state security apparatus which concerns itself with the secret activities of foreign states operating on French territory. Very little is known about the operations of this organisation. The RG are another political police agency, but their duties are focused on internal dissent, rather than the activities of outside agents.

4 Apparently the Police de l'Air et des Frontières (PAF) also have liaison officers outside Europe, notably in North Africa, French-speaking sub-Saharan Africa and South-east Asia.
5 Similar arrangements have been established for the border controls for the Channel Tunnel (ed.).

References

Anderson, M. (1989) *Policing the World*, Oxford: Clarendon Press.

Anderson, M. (1996) *Frontiers: Territory and State Formation in the Modern World*, Cambridge: Polity Press.

Anderson, M., den Boer, M., Cullen, P., Gilmore, W., Raab, C. and Walker, N. (1995) *Policing the European Union: Theory, Law and Practice*, Oxford: Clarendon Press.

Bayley, D. H. (1975) 'The Police and Political Development in Europe', in C. Tilley (ed.), *The Formation of National States in Europe*, Princeton NJ: Princeton University Press.

Bayley, D. (1992) 'Comparative Organization of the Police in English Speaking Countries', in M. Tonry and N. Morris (eds), *Modern Policing*, Vol. 15 of *Crime and Justice a Review of the Research*, Chicago: Chicago University Press.

Benyon, J. (1992) *Issues in European Police Co-operation*, Leicester University Discussion Papers in Politics, No. P92/11.

Benyon, J., Turnbull, L., Willis, A., Woodward, R., and Beck, A. (1993) *Police Cooperation in Europe: An Investigation*, Leicester: University of Leicester, Centre for the Study of Public Order.

Berger, P. and Luckmann, T. (1967) *The Social Construction of Reality: A Treatise in the Sociology of Knowledge*, London: Allen Lane, Penguin Press.

Bigo, D. (1992) *L'Europe des polices et de la sécurité intérieure*, Brussels: Complexe.

Bigo, D. (1994) 'The European Internal Security Field: Stakes and Rivalries in a Newly Developing Area of Police Intervention', in M. Anderson and M. den Boer (eds), *Policing across National Boundaries*, London: Pinter.

Bigo, D. (1996) *Polices en réseaux, l'expérience européenne*, Paris: Presses des Sciences Po.

Bigo, D. and Leveau, R. (1992) *L'Europe de la sécurité intérieure*, Paris: Institut des Hautes Etudes de Sécurité Intérieure (IHESI).

Bourdieu, P. (1990) *The Logic of Practice*, translated by Richard Nice, Cambridge: Polity Press.

Brodeur, J.-P. (1983) 'High Policing and Low Policing: Remarks about the Policing of Political Activities', *Social Problems*, Vol. 30, No. 5, pp. 507–20.

Brodeur, J.-P. (1997) *Violence and Racial Prejudice in the Context of Peacekeeping*, Ottawa: Minister of Public Works and Government Services.

Chomsky, N. (1991) *Deterring Democracy*, London: Vintage.

Clutterbuck, R. (1990) *Terrorism, Drugs and Crime in Europe after 1992*, London: Routledge.

Commonwealth Law Bulletin (1992) 'Editorial Note on United States vs Alvarez-Machain: State Sponsored Kidnapping in Lieu of Extradition', Vol. 18, pp. i–iii.

Fijnaut, C. (1991) 'Police Co-operation in Western Europe', in F. Heidensohn and M. Farrell (eds), *Crime in Europe*, London: Routledge.

Foucault, M. (1977) *Discipline and Punish: The Birth of the Prison*, translated by Alan Sheridan, London: Penguin Books.

Foucault, M. (1980) *Power/Knowledge: Selected Interviews and Other Writings 1972–1977*, C. Gordon (ed.), New York: Pantheon Books.

Foucault, M. (1989) *Sécurité, territoire et populations, résumé des cours*, Paris: Juliard.

Foucault, M. (1991) 'Politics and the Study of Discourse', in G. Burchell, C. Gordon and P. Miller (eds), *The Foucault Effect: Studies in Governmentality*, London: Harvester Wheatsheaf.

Giddens, A. (1990) *The Consequences of Modernity*, Cambridge: Polity Press.

Gleizal, J.-J., Gatti-Domenach, J. and Journes, C. (1993) *La Police. Le cas des démocraties occidentales*, Paris: Presses Universitaires de France.

Gregory, F. (1996) 'The United Nations Provision of Policing Services (CIVPOL) within the Framework of "Peacekeeping" Operations: An Analysis of the Issues', *Policing and Society*, Vol. 6, pp. 145–61.

Guyomarch, A. (1991) 'Problems of Law and Order in France in the 1980s: Politics and Professionalism', *Policing and Society*, No. 4, pp. 319–32.

Haggerty, K. and Ericson, R. (1999) 'The Militarisation of Police in the Information Age', *Journal of Political and Military Sociology*, Vol. 27 (Winter), pp. 233–55.

Harding, C., Fennell, P., Jörg, N. and Swart, B. (1995) *Criminal Justice in Europe: A Comparative Study*, Oxford: Clarendon Press.

Hurwitz, L. and Lequesne, C. (1991) *The State of the European Community: Policies, Institutions and Debates in the Transition Years*, London: Lynne Rienner.

Institut des Hautes Études de la Sécurité Intérieure (IHESI) (1992) 'Polices en Europe', *Cahiers*, No. 7, November 1991–January 1992.

Institut des Hautes Études de la Sécurité Intérieure (IHESI) (1993a) 'Gendarmeries et polices à statut militaire', *Cahiers*, No. 11, November 1992–January 1993.

Institut des Hautes Études de la Sécurité Intérieure (IHESI) (1993b) 'Systèmes de police comparés et coopération (I)', *Cahiers*, No. 13, May–July 1993.

Institut des Hautes Études de la Sécurité Intérieure (IHESI) (1993c) 'Systèmes de police comparés et coopération (II)', *Cahiers*, No. 14, August–October 1993.

Joubert, C. and Bevers, H. (1996) *Schengen Investigated: A Comparative Interpretation of the Schengen Provisions on International Police Cooperation in the Light of the European Convention on Human Rights*, The Hague: Kluwer Law Publishers.

98   *Didier Bigo*

Journés, C. (1993) 'The Structure of the French Police System: Is the French Police a National Force?', *International Journal of the Sociology of Law*, Vol. 21, pp. 281–7.

Katzenstein, P. (1990) *West Germany's Internal Security Policy: State and Violence in the 1970s and 1980s*, Occasional Paper No. 28, Ithaca NY: Cornell University, Centre for International Studies.

Katzenstein, P. (1996) *Cultural Norms and National Security: Police and Military in Postwar Japan*, Ithaca NY: Cornell University Press.

Keohane, R. (1989) *International Institutions and State Power*, Boulder CO: Westview Press.

Keohane, R. and Hoffman, S. (1991) *The New European Community: Decision-making and Institutional Change*, Boulder CO: Westview Press.

Keohane, R. and Nye, J. (1972) *Transnational Relations and World Politics*, Cambridge MA: Harvard University Press.

Lacroix, B. (1985) 'Ordre politique et ordre social', pp. 469–565 in J. Leca and M. Grawitz (eds), *Traité de science politique*, Vol. 1, Paris: Presses Universitaires de France.

Luhmann, N. (1995) *Social Systems*, translated by John Bednarz with Dirk Baecker, foreword by Eva M. Knodt, Stanford CT: Stanford University Press.

McIntosh, M. (1975) *The Organisation of Crime*, London: Macmillan Press.

Marx, G. (1981) 'Ironies of Social Control: Authorities as Contributors to Deviance through Escalation, Non-Enforcement and Covert Facilitation', *Social Problems*, Vol. 28, No. 3, pp. 221–46.

Monar, J. and Morgan R. (1995) *The Third Pillar of the European Union: Cooperation in the Fields of Justice and Home Affairs*, Brussels: Interuniversity Press.

Monjardet, D. (1985) 'A la recherche du travail policier', *Sociologie du Travail*, Vol. 27, No. 4, pp. 391–407.

Monjardet, D. and Lévy, R. (1995) 'Undercover Policing in France', in C. Fijnaut and G. Marx (eds), *Undercover: Police Surveillance in Comparative Perspective*, The Hague: Kluwer.

Nadelmann, E. A. (1993a) *Cops across Borders: The Internationalization of US Criminal Law Enforcement*, University Park PA: Pennsylvania State University Press.

Nadelmann, E. (1993b) 'US Police Activities in Europe', in C. Fijnaut (ed.), *The Internationalization of Police Cooperation in Western Europe*, Gouda Quint: Kluwer.

Porta, Donatela Della (1995) *Social Movements, Political Violence and the State*, Cambridge: Cambridge University Press.

Quermonne, J. L. (1992) 'Trois lectures du traité de Maastricht: essai d'analyse comparative', *Revue Française de Science Politique*, Vol. 42, No. 5, October, pp. 311–45.

Reiner, R. (1992) *The Politics of the Police*, 2nd edition, Toronto: University of Toronto Press.

Tilley, C. (1985) 'War Making and State Making as Organized Crime', in P. Evans, D. Rueschemeyer and T. Skocpol (eds), *Bringing the State Back In*, Cambridge: Cambridge University Press.

Sheptycki, J. W. E. (1995) 'Transnational Policing and the Makings of a Post-modern State', *British Journal of Criminology*, Vol. 35, No. 4, pp. 613–35.

Sheptycki, J. W. E. (1996) 'Law Enforcement, Justice and Democracy in the Transnational Arena: Reflections on the War on Drugs', *International Journal of the Sociology of Law*, Vol. 24, No. 1, pp. 61–75.

Sheptycki, J. W. E. (1997a) 'Faire la police dans la Manche: l'évolution de la co-opération transfrontalière (1968–1996)', *Cultures et Conflits*, Édition Spécial: *Contrôles: Frontières-Identités: Les enjeux autour de l'immigration et de l'asile*, Vols. 26/27, pp. 93–123.

Sheptycki, J. W. E. (1997b) 'Transnationalism, Crime Control and the European State System: A Review of the Literature', *International Criminal Justice Review*, Vol. 7, pp. 130–40.

Sheptycki, J. W. E. (1998a) 'The Global Cops Cometh: Reflections on Transnationalization, Knowledge Work and Policing Subculture', *British Journal of Sociology*, Vol. 49, No. 1, pp. 57–74.

Sheptycki, J. W. E. (1998b) 'Review of Schengen Investigated', *International Journal of Evidence and Proof*, Vol. 1, No. 4, pp. 246–9.

Sheptycki, J. W. E. (1998c) 'Policing, Postmodernism and Transnationalisation', *British Journal of Criminology*, Vol. 38, No. 3, pp. 485–503.

Sheptycki, J. W. E. (1999) 'Political Culture and Structures of Social Control: Police Related Scandal in Low Countries in Comparative Perspective', *Policing and Society*, Vol. 9, No. 1, pp. 1–31.

Singer, M. and Wildavsky, A. (1993) *The Real World Order: Zones of Peace and Zones of Turmoil*, Chatham NJ: Chatham House.

Sivanandan, A. (1993) 'Beyond Statewatching', in T. Bunyan (ed.), *Statewatching the New Europe: A Handbook on the European State*, London: Statewatch.

Streeck, W. and Schmitter, P. C. (1991) 'From National Corporatism to Transnational Pluralism: Organised Interests in the Single European Market', *Politics and Society*, Vol. 19, pp. 133–64.

Tannenbaum, F. (1938) *Crime and the Community*, New York: Columbia University Press.

Veyne, P. (1984) *Writing History: Essays on Epistemology*, translated by Mina Moore-Rinvolucri, Manchester: Manchester University Press.

Veyne, P. (1990) *Bread and Circuses: Historical Sociology and Political Pluralism*, translated by Brian Pearce, London: Allen Lane, Penguin Press.

Walker, N. (1994) 'European Integration and European Policing: A Complex Relationship', in M. Anderson and M. den Boer (eds), *Policing across National Boundaries*, London: Pinter.

Waltz, K. N. (1993) 'The Emerging Structure of International Politics', in *International Security*, Vol. 18, No. 2, pp. 44–7.

4 Private criminality as a matter of international concern

Frank Gregory

Introduction

This chapter seeks to examine how actions by individuals, for private gain, become classified as crimes of international significance and how states address the problems of transnational law enforcement. It draws partly on the growing literature on international criminal law (on broader usage of international law see Slaughter et al. 1998), and on the historical studies of three early foci for transnational law enforcement: the control of piracy, the slave trade and drug trafficking. It also analyses the development of international crime control concerns by the United Nations (UN) and the European Union (EU).

The chapter aims to provide a general understanding of international policing regimes. In previous studies (Gregory 1995 and 1996) some of these issues were addressed in the context of police, as commonly understood, working outside their national boundaries. For example, as civilian police (CIVPOL) units in UN peacekeeping operations or when police officers are invited to carry out or assist criminal investigations on the territory of another state. However, while preparing this contribution, it was evident that a broader construction of the practice of transnational policing could be developed. International policing, for the purposes of this chapter, refers to the involvement of state public bodies both in national criminal justice systems and others (such as the armed forces) that can be authorised and tasked to help in criminal justice matters in respect of private criminality involving more than one state. This definition can therefore cover activities in support of crime suppression treaties, for example, the use of warships to intercept and detain ships carrying slaves. It can also cover judicial co-operation actions in support of treaties establishing processes to aid the control of transnational crime, principally those relating to extradition, mutual legal assistance and the specification of common schedules of offences.

Drawing on international criminal law (particularly Dugard and van den Wyngaert 1996) allows us to examine crime in its international context in a more detached manner than working from speculative quantifications of the problems or the over-dramatisation of global Mafias and global crime conspiracies. International law requires us to consider crime in terms of degrees of severity of offence and thus in the levels of response that may be required of states. It also provides a clear threshold for calling an anti-social act a crime. That is to say, what is alleged to be a crime must be established in law as a crime. It will be argued that international law currently provides three expressions of the degree of severity with which states regard particular offences by individuals.

Firstly, there are the offences within the terms of the legal regime covering war crimes and crimes against humanity. Secondly, there are certain other individual criminal acts which attract such universal condemnation as to render the perpetrator '*hostis humani generis*, an enemy of all mankind' (Malenczuk 1997: 114). The crimes of piracy and slave trading are well established in this category. Thirdly, there is the growing category of offences whose characteristics transcend the domestic law sphere by involving actions in two or more states' territories and where the conclusion of an international law prohibition or suppression instrument is held to be the appropriate response, for example, the Council of Europe Convention on Terrorism (1977) and the United Nations (Vienna) Convention on Drug Trafficking (1988).

It will not be the intention of this chapter to argue that the category of 'crimes against humanity' should now include the drug trafficker or the paedophile, although some politicians may so argue. Rather it will explore both possible extensions to the category of *hostis humani generis* and the increased use of crime control treaties. A further advantage of tracking the development of international legal instruments is that it produces a longer temporal reference period, avoiding an over-concentration on the post-1989 period. In tracing the development of the treaties relating to private criminality the chapter can also update Nadelmann's authoritative analysis published in 1990 (and see also McDonald (ed.) 1997). Nadelmann's study of global prohibition regimes and the evolution of norms in international society focuses on norms which prohibit, both in the international and domestic criminal laws of states, the involvement of state and non-actors in particular activities. He specifies acts such as piracy, slavery, trafficking in slaves, counterfeiting of national currencies, hijacking of aircraft, trafficking in women and children for the purposes of prostitution, and trafficking in controlled psychoactive substances (Nadelmann 1990: 479).

Nadelmann also identified two characteristics of this process which are central to the concerns of this chapter. These are that the substance of these norms and the enforcement processes are 'institutionalized in global prohibition regimes' and that only 'crimes that evidence a strong transnational dimension have become the subject of international prohibition regimes' (pp. 479, 481). Alongside the international criminal law classification of crimes this chapter will also draw upon Nadelmann's identification (p. 484) of five evolutionary stages in the development of prohibition regimes. These are, in brief: (1) activity lawful, (2) activity redefined as a problem, (3) agitation for suppression and criminalisation, (4) activity becomes criminal offence and (5) hopefully, activity significantly decreases.

This chapter does not cover those acts of individuals which, although constituting internationally recognised crimes, have been considered open to a 'political factors' defence. The problems of developing international legal instruments to specify individual criminality in respect of terrorist acts can be illustrated by reference to the limited progress made since the UN adopted General Assembly Resolution (GAR) 40/61 in December 1985. This resolution unconditionally condemned 'as criminal all acts, methods and practice of terrorism' (Zmeeski and Tarabin 1996: 83). Yet by 1998 the only instrument adopted (GAR 52/164) for signature was the highly crime specific UN International Convention for the Suppression of Terrorist Bombings (UN 1998b).

The chapter commences with a discussion of selected writings on international criminal law in order to establish some basic meanings of terminology and scope. It then reviews the prohibition and suppression regimes directed against piracy, slavery and slave trading. These were the first two activities for private gain by individuals to be recognised as universal crimes and resulted in transnational responses. This is followed by a consideration of drug trafficking. The efforts to control drug-trafficking are especially significant in the contemporary period because they have become linked to much broader concerns such as money-laundering, multi-activity organised crime (crime as business) and corruption.

These reviews are followed by a comparative analysis of the growing recognition of crime as a matter of concern in two politically important fora, the United Nations and the European Union. As with the historical examples, global recognition of an activity as a crime tends to require the active involvement of the major states and thus criminalisation reflects dominant interests, political, economic or moral. In the case of the UN's response, attention is drawn to the current focus on a particular form of criminality, organised crime, a contested term, but nevertheless a preoccupation in the USA and Europe. The efforts to establish common standards for the prohibition and suppression of corruption are considered next. It is argued that the concern with corruption is part of a recognition that policing transnational crime requires that some attention be paid to the capacity of criminals to place themselves beyond the reach of the law by the use of corruption. The chapter concludes with the question of whether the new International Criminal Court might be able to exercise any jurisdiction over private criminality.

International criminal law and the scope for transnational policing

The scope and dimensions of international criminal law (ICL) are a matter on which there is a spectrum of opinions among eminent lawyers. Key contributions have been assembled in Dugard and van den Wyngaert's edited volume *International Criminal Law and Procedure* (1996) and this section draws on two of those contributions. Georg Schwarzenberger (1950), the author of a classic text on international law (5th edition 1967) and then a Professor of Law at London University, represents what Dugard and van den Wyngaert call the restrictive, positivist (or Hobbesian) perspective. This emphasises international law working within an international system dominated by state interest. By contrast, M. Cherif Bassiouni, who has achieved eminence both in America and through the International Law Commission and, latterly, through chairing the 1998 international conference which produced the Rome Statute for the new International Criminal Court, reflects, in his writings, what Dugard and van den Wyngaert (1996: xiii) identify as the use of a 'wider framework of jurisprudential inquiry, in which contemporary idealist and sociological theories of law [produce] a less cautious assessment of international criminal law'.

Because he could identify six different meanings for international criminal law Schwarzenberger, writing in 1950, felt that its status as a technical term still had to be clarified. However, among his six interpretations of international criminal law one does find important statements of scope and process. These are, firstly, the territorial scope of national law, that is how far any state seeks to encompass crimes with a foreign element, with the caveat that actual exercises of jurisdiction (or policing) must conform to a definitive prohibitive rule of international law, which is that states only have jurisdiction over their own territory or overseas possessions and their 'flagged' ships or aircraft, when the latter are not within another state's jurisdiction. This rule is perhaps the most significant limitation on the practice of transnational policing. Secondly, the requirement for national law to reflect international prohibition or suppression conventions, for example, with regard to the crimes of piracy and drug trafficking. Thirdly, a corollary of the second point, that states have an obligation to at least attempt to suppress such acts as piracy or drug trafficking or risk being considered an 'outlaw' state. Fourthly, that treaties or conventions give rise to national obligations in terms of the processes of transnational policing through extradition and mutual legal assistance requirements. If there was to be an international criminal law more akin to national criminal law then, for Schwarzenberger, it would only protect the highest values and interests of states and encompass acts 'which strike at the very roots of society' (Schwarzenberger quoted in Dugard and van den Wyngaert 1996: 13).

By contrast Bassiouni (1974: 68, 70, 85) postulates a changed scenario in which international society has evolved to a position where the 'world community has come to require of its participants a greater degree of conformity and compliance with certain minimum standards of behaviour for the attainment of its perceived goals of collective and personal security'. Thus, for Bassiouni, ICL is one of the strategies to achieve these goals. He sees ICL as being derived from both co-operation to enforce national criminal law and from the criminal aspects of international law which cover, *inter alia*, war crimes and 'common crimes against internationally protected interests'. These he defines as 'acts committed by individuals or small groups in furtherance of private or pecuniary but non-governmental interests which constitute a violation of specific international criminal law proscriptions'. The minimum requirement for states in these cases is to prosecute or extradite. This contention does seem to describe much of the current efforts of states in developing international prohibition or suppression agreements.

Moreover, Bassiouni (ibid: 85–6), in this context, sets out seven characteristics that are common to such crimes. These are:

1   The criminalised conduct is individual conduct even when committed by small groups;
2   the motive for the conduct is private or personal but non-governmental;
3   it causes harm to persons or private interests;
4   it involves criminal activities spanning more than one state in its planning or commission;

5   the interest it affects is a matter of concern to all or a substantial
     number of states and consequently states share an interest in pre-
     venting, controlling and suppressing such conduct;
6   to accomplish that result international co-operation is essential;
7   the conduct in question is usually a municipal crime under national
     criminal law.

It can readily be agreed that the characteristics, set out by Bassiouni
above, are congruent with the recent and contemporary treatment of
problems such as drug trafficking and organised crime by states. Additionally, the stages of action by which activities are criminalised, identified by Bassiouni, are broadly consistent with Nadelmann's (1990)
analysis.

Reflecting on the positions of Schwarzenberger and Bassiouni, one
can see considerable similarities with regard to established international criminal law, what lawyers would call the *lex lata* position.
That is to say, international criminal law reflects a non-supranational
prohibition regime as its enforcement is dependent upon the actions
of states. This point is echoed by Nadelmann, to wit: 'An international criminal law is most potent . . . when it reflects not just self-
interest but a broadly acknowledged moral obligation' (Nadelmann
1990: 490).

However, Bassiouni also believes (1974: 94) that attention to what
lawyers call the *de lege ferenda* or law development process, could
address the weaknesses of a state-centric system which has 'no criminological policy' and 'no system to ensure compliance by enforcing
agents'. In particular he advocates a codification of international criminal law and the establishment of an international criminal court. Thus
his position is partly an early anticipation of the more proactive stance
of the UN on international crime occurring after the mid-1980s. The
late and post-Cold War concerns of major states about crime threats
in emergent security agendas, in particular the hegemonic influence of
the United States, loom large here.

Piracy

Whilst the categorisation of the pirate as 'the common enemy of
mankind' by Alberico Gentili in the sixteenth century may suggest a
long history of international condemnation of this form of private
criminality, Pugh (1994: 80) has reminded us that some societies and
states have given social and political recognition to piracy. Moreover,
in past conflicts, maritime powers such as Britain and France have

been prepared to give particular pirates lawful status by letters of *marque* and reprisal, commissioning their vessels and crews as privateers or private warships flying national flags and acting in support of national belligerent policy.

It is instructive to review some of the recent historical and legal writings on piracy (e.g. Nadelmann 1990; Lubbock 1993; Rubin 1997; Starkey et al. 1997) because they help us to deconstruct piracy into categories that aid an understanding of the problem and reveal the limitations of international responses. Anderson (1997: 88) provides a valuable three-part classification of piracy:

> Parasitic – a function of the volume of trade and the degree of protection of trade available;
>
> Episodic – lack of economic alternatives for maritime communities;
>
> Intrinsic – integral to 'state' or societal activities – Vikings, Etruscans, Barbary corsairs, Malay states and Persian Gulf states in the eighteenth and nineteenth centuries, or where a state was unwilling or unable to exercise national jurisdiction, e.g. China in the nineteenth century.

Geographically the depredations of many pirate groups were practised in coastal or even riverine waters. For example, Murray has drawn attention to the Chinese pirate communities which existed between 1750 and 1850. He noted that in Kwantung province the pirate confederation consisted of seven fleets (c. 2,000 junks) and 50,000–70,000 pirates. This pirate fleet was so fearsome that, according to Murray, scarcely a junk dared leave port without first paying the pirates protection money against attacks. Having gained control of the waterways the pirates next moved into the interior where they extorted considerable sums in the form of semi-annual payments from the villages and towns, 'burning with impunity those that refused to pay' (Murray 1997: 49).

The recent studies of pre-twentieth-century piracy agree on the strategies that brought piracy down to a minimal level. These were: use of the naval forces of the major European powers and the USA, growing state power to control coastal areas in the Americas and the Caribbean and the process of European colonisation and establishment of protectorates. For example, the control of piracy in the Persian Gulf and in the waters around Malaya was greatly aided by the expansion of British political and naval power in those regions. Crucially, the exercise of naval power in controlling piracy was not confined to the high seas, but was extended to include coastal actions and landings.

Needless to say, the latter activities by major powers would be considered unacceptable today.

Piracy is now proscribed by both established principles of customary international law and treaty law. Schwarzenberger identifies two key principles of customary international law which have been developed from reciprocal treaties between states in the Middle Ages (Schwarzenberger 1950: 266–9). These are, firstly, that every state is under an obligation to suppress piracy in its territorial jurisdiction; secondly, that in the interests of the freedom of the high seas, any state can assume jurisdiction on the high seas over pirate ships because pirates are presumed not to be under the sovereignty of any state. However, Rubin's meticulous study (1997) shows that even arriving at these proscriptions has been a long and problematic process because of issues relating to both state practice and lack of precision in applications of the term 'piracy'. Rubin is also very concerned about the true legal standing of enforcement actions against piracy on the high seas and he suggests that there may only be 'universal jurisdiction to enforce and to adjudicate in some places and in some very narrow circumstance' (p. 394).

The most recent treaty law is contained in Article 101 of the UN Law of the Sea Convention (1982) which defines the offence in the following terms:

(a) any illegal acts of violence or detention, or any act of depredation committed for private ends by the crew or passengers of a private ship or a private aircraft, and directed;

   (i) on the high seas against another ship or aircraft or against persons or property on board such an aircraft;
   (ii) against a ship or, aircraft, persons or property in a place outside the jurisdiction of any State;

(b) any act of voluntary participation in the operation of a ship or aircraft with knowledge of facts making it a pirate ship or aircraft;
(c) any act of initiating or of intentionally facilitating an act as described in sub-paragraph (a) or (b).

(as cited in Pugh 1994: 81–2)

Because of the 'private ends' qualification, incidents such as the Palestinian terrorist seizure of the cruise ship *Achille Lauro* in 1985 come within the scope of separate treaty law, the 1988 Rome Convention for the Suppression of Unlawful Acts Against the Safety of Maritime Navigation (see Ronzitti 1990).

In the early 1990s piracy seemed to be re-emerging as a threat and
Britain and Russia were reported as calling for some form of international naval action in the Asia–Pacific region (Pugh 1994: 80). However, it has been pointed out that 'an estimated 80 per cent of so called
"piracy" is not piracy on the high seas as legally defined, but raiding in
territorial waters' (p. 83). Thus whilst in the last century the pirate on
the high seas may have seemed the epitome of an enemy of all mankind, the modern pirate is more typically akin to bandits on land.

Vagg has carried out a detailed study of contemporary piracy in
South-east Asia and his findings echo those of Pugh (Vagg 1995).
Firstly, many of the 'piracy' incidents he analysed took place in, or
very close to, territorial waters and, hence, are really just crimes against
national criminal laws. For example, Vagg found that in the Riau area
between Malaysia, Singapore and Indonesia, between 1990 and 1992
there was a tenfold increase in 'piracy'. However, there seems to have
been a general consensus from the flag states of victim vessels, neigh-
bouring states and the International Maritime Bureau that enhanced
local law enforcement co-operation could control the problem, much
of which was believed to lie within Indonesian jurisdiction. Chalk came
to similar conclusions in his study of the Indonesian region (Chalk
1998) and he also pointed out that many incidents took place in harbours and anchorages. This was certainly true in 1995, as 16 out of 17
reported incidents took place in Jakarta's territorial waters and were
not piracy in any formal international law sense but what the International Maritime Bureau classifies as 'low-level armed robbery.' Thus
much of contemporary piracy is, by virtue of its common location in
harbours, territorial waters or near territorial waters, more a matter
for routine national law enforcement which can be of variable quality
depending on the political will and/or resources of particular states.

The slave trade

Whilst the pirate had few defenders, at least in the abstract, the slave
trader was for several centuries seen as a legitimate entrepreneur and
trader whose commodity was human bodies rather than goods or
money. It required a significant shift in moral attitudes before the
slave trader was seen in the same light as the pirate. This point about
moral motivations is made forcibly by Nadelmann and he also reminds us that the 'crusade required not only the outlawing of the trade
but also of the institution of slavery' (Nadelmann 1990: 493).

The recent study of slavery by Thomas (1997; see also Lloyd 1968)
provides a valuable source from which to reconstruct the linkages

between the attempts to outlaw the trade, the judicial process problems and the law enforcement difficulties. Such an exercise is very useful for demonstrating the inherent problems in transnational law enforcement and the time it takes to change social and political attitudes. Discussions about the propriety of the slave trade, at legislative level, did not commence in America, Britain and France until the years 1788–91 and the main slave trade (from West Africa to the Americas) continued until the 1870s. Moreover, in terms of the slave traffic between East Africa and Arabia, the last reported capture of a slave dhow was carried out by HMS *Cornflower* in 1922 (Lubbock 1993: 2).

Schwarzenberger considers that the most celebrated case of international criminal law becoming part of international treaty law is the 'gradual assimilation by means of bilateral and multilateral treaties of slave trading to piracy' (Schwarzenberger 1950: 23–4). An important feature was the recognition by the anti-slavery states that modifications to international law depended on the free consent of every sovereign state. Where bilateral or multilateral jurisdiction was provided for it only applied to questions of adjudication to determine that vessels were slave traders. Criminal jurisdiction over owners and crews was a matter for each state according to its national criminal laws.

Radical but unadopted proposals were made at a meeting of the European Great Powers at Aix-la-Chapelle in 1818. These included proposals for an international right of search of suspect slave ships. The Congress also proposed 'the vigilant superintendence of an armed and international police on the coast of West Africa . . . [further] . . . To render such a police either legal or effective in its objective, it must be established under the sanction, and by the authority, of all civilised states' (Thomas 1997: 592). The vision was of a police with universal jurisdiction, but such an aim was too far in advance of the actual or potential level of state political will. Thus anti-piracy action was undertaken at the national and bilateral level.

A series of important national initiatives occurred in the period 1818–30. In 1818 France declared the slave trade illegal. In 1820 the US President was empowered to cause any of the armed vessels of the United States to be employed to cruise on any of the coasts of the United States or territories thereof, or off the coasts of Africa or elsewhere to seize American slavers. A further attempt to develop multilateral action was the 1841 quintuple Treaty (Britain, France, Austria, Russia and Prussia). This declared the slave trade to be piracy and authorised any warship to search every merchant vessel belonging to one of the signatory states, although France refused to ratify this treaty.

By this treaty, the signatory states gained an exceptional jurisdiction over suspected slave vessels. But the signatory states recognised that the consent of a wider number of states would only be achieved over a longer time. The process could, however, as Schwarzenberger notes 'be prompted by bilateral and multilateral action' (Schwarzenberger 1950: 25–6). Moreover the British specifically recognised the limitations of international authority over non-signatory states. Referring to the case of Turkey, the Secretary to the Board of Admiralty wrote, in December 1845, that 'in the absence of a treaty with the Porte it would be illegal for British naval forces in the Black Sea to detain Turkish vessels conveying slaves from Georgia to Circassia' (ibid). Significantly, this recognition came from the dominant naval power. Alongside the elaboration of this legal apparatus there was a growth in European-American naval anti-slavery patrols between West Africa and the Americas. In 1845 Britain had 38 ships on anti-slavery patrol, France 28, America between three and eight and Portugal nine. A significant bilateral treaty was that of 1861 between America and Britain granting mutual search powers to each other's warships.

It is generally accepted that the slave trade between Africa and the Americas was ended by about 1871, after the colonisation of West Africa and the abolition of slavery in the American south. But this still left several decades of work by the Royal Navy, to control the East Africa–Arabia slave trade. Thus, if we take 1788 as the start of serious government-level efforts to control the African slave trade, and the dhow seizure by HMS *Cornflower* in 1922 as the end of concerted action against the trade, this totals a period of approximately 140 years of effort. What are the lessons for current efforts against newly identified forms of international crime? Firstly, achieving a moral and legal consensus was a long process. Secondly, enforcement depended mainly on one naval power, in the historical instance considered here, Britain. Thirdly, both ends of the trade needed to be subjected to controls – abolition of slavery in the receiving states and imposition of colonial power in the sending areas. Fourthly, the policing actions were confined to the sea transport of African slaves.

The anti-slavery prohibition regime is the only regime to exhibit all five of Nadelmann's evolutionary stages. He also identified the following factors of significance about the anti-slavery regime: it was the first to be institutionalised by treaty law; the first instance of the key role of moral impulses; the first to criminalise a particular commodity; and, lastly, the first to criminalise all aspects of production, sale and use. Nadelmann also made the cautionary point that the prohibition regime did not encompass other forms of slavery like bonded labour, and that actual slave trading continued to exist in Africa itself (Nadelmann 1990: 497). Additionally, the suppression of both piracy and slavery could, in large part, take advantage of the policing opportunities provided by the high seas for the exercise of extra-territorial jurisdiction. It will become apparent that, as the international crime agenda develops in scope, this medium for international policing becomes much less significant.

Drug trafficking and agenda broadening

The frustration of the attempts to control drug trafficking provides a very significant example 'of the capacity of a transnational activity to resist the combined efforts of governments' (Nadelmann 1990: 512). Indeed, in observing the leading role played by the United States in the anti-drug crusade and the congruence with the abortive alcohol prohibition period in America, one can point to clear examples of criminalisation of commodities stimulating the growth of clandestine markets. This has been an important factor in the contemporary broadening of the development of international criminal law prohibition and suppression regimes to encompass money laundering, organised crime and corruption. The 1997 UN International Drug Control Programme clearly sets out these issues as seen from the perspective of the United Nations:

> Large scale international movements of cocaine and heroin are almost entirely controlled by transnational organized crime groups, for whom drugs are consequently a primary source of revenue. Over the last 20 years, drug trafficking organisations have increasingly diversified into other forms of criminal activities in order to protect their primary interests, such as arms trafficking, money laundering and penetration of the legal economic, political, and administrative sectors.
>
> (UNDCP 1997: 133)

In its development up until now, the regime to control the use of, and traffic in, narcotic and psychotropic substances has passed through all the stages identified by Nadelmann (see also Chatterjee 1980) but, as noted above, it is not fulfilling the fifth stage hope of withering under the effects of criminalisation. The basic principles of international narcotics law were laid down in the International Opium Convention of 1912 (the Hague Convention). The Convention's principles were: legal control of raw opium production and distribution; gradual suppression of opium smoking; limitation of manufactured narcotics (cocaine and morphine) to medical and legitimate needs and subjection of manufacturers and traders to a system of permits and regulations. By World War II international co-operation was founded on domestic supervision based on evolving international law, the international supervision of domestic control via the Permanent Central Opium Board, the League of Nations Advisory Committee on the Traffic in Opium and Other Dangerous Drugs and limited moves towards true transnational control.

When the United Nations was established in 1945 it continued the League of Nations' work in developing the drug control and suppression regime (see Gregg 1964). The bases, in international law, of inter-state anti-narcotic co-operation are currently: the 1961 Single Convention on Narcotic Drugs (codifying conventions passed between 1912 and 1953) and the 1971 Convention on Psychotropic Substances. As a basis for state action and co-operation the 1961 Single Convention provides, firstly, under Article 4, that signatories must take all necessary steps to limit production of designated drugs exclusively to medical and scientific uses and, secondly, that they must enact appropriate criminal offences and penalties (Articles 35–6).

Thus the evolutionary decades of emerging international law on narcotics control produced an 'indirect approach' to the problem because responsibility for control rested firmly on the proper exercise of *domestic* jurisdiction by states. However, such a system contains an inherent weakness which was recognised in the Final Report in 1967 of the Permanent Narcotics Control Board. The Report concluded that the 'greatest obstacles to further progress in international narcotics control are to be found in territories with a "drug economy", i.e. those whose economies depend on the sale of opium for illicit purposes or on that of coca leaves'. However, a similar comment could also be made about the problems of effective national controls with regard to the production of synthetic drugs (psychotropic substances) in the developed states.

In order that transnational control could assume a greater prominence the scale of the social problems of drug abuse needed political recognition as a major public policy issue. By the end of the 1960s such a recognition occurred in states with the capacity to influence the treatment of the issue at the international level. In September 1968, the then US presidential candidate, Richard Nixon, said in a speech at Anaheim, California, that he would, as President, move against drugs source areas and the traffic in drugs. The concept of a 'war' on drugs has been a domestic and international policy theme continued by successive US presidents ever since. European recognition of a rising drugs problem was marked, in 1971, by the establishment of the Council of Europe's Pompidou Group, following a French initiative. By the 1980s this international crime issue had even crossed the East–West ideological divide. The USSR had begun to admit a domestic drug abuse problem and that the traffic needed controlling. In the summer of 1987 the Russian Health Minister told the UN Conference on Drug Abuse and Illicit Trafficking that there had been a 'certain increase' in drug abuse in the USSR and that it caused concern and needed 'resolute state measures' (*The Independent* 1 July 1987). Whereas, in 1984, the official figures gave the number of registered addicts in the USSR as 2,400 by '1987 officials admitted to 123,000 drug abusers, including 46,000 registered addicts' (Galeotti 1993: 771). East–West bilateral action swiftly followed with Britain and the USSR concluding an inter-customs agency mutual aid agreement. This led in April 1988, to Operation Diplomat through which British customs seized £10 million worth of Afghan cannabis following a joint Anglo-Soviet operation.

In addition to a growing East–West consensus, pressures for enhanced international law enforcement came also from the drugs source countries who are concerned at the domestic instability caused by the economic power of the drugs traffickers. As in the case of developing controls on the slave trade, both ends of the drugs trade were in a position to support enhanced law enforcement measures. At the Annual UN Drugs Conference in 1987, Señor Parejo Gonzales, the Colombian Minister of Justice, who had survived an assassination attempt by drugs traffickers, described himself as 'a symbol of the unrelenting and inflexible position the international community must adopt in pursuit of the drugs Mafia' (*The Times* 17 January 1987 and 3 February 1987). By the end of the 1980s drug trafficking topped the list of internationally recognised crimes and states were prepared to contemplate a significant development in their international legal obligations. That development was to be enshrined in the 1988 UN (Vienna) Convention against the Illicit Traffic in Narcotic Drugs and Psychotropic Substances.

The international legal instruments referred to above come within the third category of expressions in international law of the degree of severity accorded by states to offences committed by individuals. That is where the characteristics of the offences transcend state boundaries for the commission of the offences and in 'spill-over' effects. But, as yet, in this category the perpetrators are not seen as either akin to 'war criminals' or as *enemies of all mankind*. In this context the 1988 United

Nations Convention Against Illicit Traffic in Narcotic Drugs and Psychotropic Substances (The Vienna Convention – UN ECOSOC 1988) is an important statement of general principles regarding the development of international criminal law and an important source of legal authority for actions to control drug trafficking. The preamble expresses the rationale for the Convention in the following terms:

- scale and rising trend threatening 'the health and welfare of human beings and adversely [affecting] the economic, cultural and political foundations of society';
- the links between illicit traffic and other related organised criminal activities which undermine the legitimate economies and threaten the stability, security and sovereignty of States;
- the illicit traffic is an international criminal activity, the suppression of which demands urgent attention and the highest priority;
- the illicit traffic generates large financial profits and wealth enabling international criminal organisations to penetrate, contaminate and corrupt the structures of government, legitimate commercial and financial barriers and society at all levels.

The latter part of the preamble formally expresses the increasing scope of the international crime agenda in areas such as corruption and financial crime and a recognition of the 'grey area' between licit and illicit activities.

Within this Convention there are four specific crime control measures that emphasise the significance of this instrument of international criminal law. Firstly, Article 3 which requires states to establish, at the national level, a common schedule of offences and sanctions. Secondly, Article 4 on jurisdiction requires states to try their own nationals for offences under the Convention, even if committed outside their national territory, in cases where a state chooses not to extradite the offender. Thirdly, Article 11 gives international approval to the use of 'controlled deliveries' where domestic legal systems so allow. Fourthly, Article 17 on the 'Illicit Traffic by Sea' takes full advantage of the freedom of high seas from national jurisdictions to follow the crime control precedents of piracy and the slave trade.

Under Article 17(3) warships, military aircraft or other government service ships or aircraft, for example, the US Coastguard or UK Customs and Excise may take actions against suspect vessels of another state under the conditions set out next. Firstly, Article 17(3) has to be used to obtain authorisation from the vessel's flag state. Thereafter, the flag state giving authorisation can permit the requesting states to board, search, seize and detain with respect to vessel, cargo and persons (Article 17(4) a–c). While the Vienna Convention's provisions regarding the interception of vessels on the high seas suspected of drug smuggling may sound permissive, the due process requirements can, at times, be quite restrictive. For example, at Bristol Crown Court, in February 1999, Judge John Foley ruled that HM Customs had abused due process in respect of British, Maltese and international law in the seizure (100 miles off the Portuguese coast) of the Maltese-registered, British-crewed MV *Simon de Danser* by HMS *York* in May 1997. While 4,128 kg of cannabis resin with an estimated street value of £14.5 million was found, the judge ended the trial before the jury was even sworn in. Among the procedural errors cited, the judge noted the fact that flag-state permission to intercept was obtained from the Director of the Maltese Maritime Authority whereas only the Maltese Attorney-General could give official approval (*The Times* 5 February 1999).

Drug traffickers are now prompting governmental responses similar to the very active suppression of pirates and slavers in the nineteenth century. The US in particular has tended to act as though drug traffickers could be treated as 'the common enemies of mankind'. In certain cases the US has claimed and practised extra-territorial jurisdiction. Rayfuse (1993) has contended that in 'the fight against international crime, where the interests of the United States are at stake, the US Supreme Court has confirmed that the rule of the jungle reigns' (cited in Dugard and van den Wyngaert 1996: 265). She illustrated this point with several cases, the most notable of which is the 1990 case of Dr Humbero Alvarez-Machain. Alvarez-Machain was abducted in Mexico and brought to Texas for arrest and trial on the charge of complicity in the murder of a US Drugs Enforcement Agency official. No request was made by the United States to Mexico for Machain's extradition. Rather, in April 1990, a number of armed men, acting on behalf of the DEA, broke into Machain's office in Guadalajara, Mexico, seized him and put him on a plane bound for El Paso, Texas where, on arrival, he was arrested by DEA agents and taken to Los Angeles to stand trial.

The Supreme Court ruled (US v. Alvarez-Machain, 1992) by six to three that there had been no violation of the US–Mexico Extradition Treaty. A similar case, Verdugo-Urquidez occurred in 1986. When the case came before the Supreme Court the majority upheld the abduction. The US Chief Justice even refused 'to interpret the [extradition] Treaty in accordance with the principles of customary international law relating to the exercise of police power in the territory of another State' (Dugard and van den Wyngaert 1996: 270). Bassiouni and Blakesley (1992), citing an even more high-profile case, US v. Noriega

(1990), expressed concerns over one of the US objectives in the Panama invasion as being to 'seize General Noriega to face federal drugs charges in the United States' (p. 102). This is a case made all the more bizarre by the revelations that US intelligence agencies had, in the past, turned a blind eye to Noriega's illegal activities when he was perceived as politically useful. This form of unilateral action, referred to as a 'kind of judicial imperialism' (Anderson, J. B. 1991: 446), may be counteracted if states can achieve a consensus on the categories of crimes and control measures that need to be formulated through international law responses. In the meantime, a broad suppression goal was agreed in the Political Declaration from the conclusion of the June 1998 UN Drugs Summit. The Declaration contained a commitment to eliminate or significantly reduce illicit cultivation of opium poppy, coca bush and cannabis plant by the year 2008 (Arlacchi 1998: 42).

The formulation of contemporary crime control agendas – The UN and the EU compared

By comparing the crime agendas of these two organisations it is possible to demonstrate that the effects of globalisation in the contemporary period produce a much more rapid and broader emergence of crime issues at the international level than was the case in the previous centuries.

Clark (1996) provides the most detailed guide to the evolution of the UN's crime control agenda and the following sections are partly based on his study. Whilst the UN has, since its foundation in 1945, always considered matters to do with the prevention of crime and the treatment of offenders, Clark noted that crime items were treated very 'perfunctorily' in the Economic and Social Council (ECOSOC) up to 1983. However, the UN's specialist forum, the UN Congresses on the Prevention of Crime and the Treatment of Offenders (UNCPCTO) began to treat certain developments in criminality as warranting international attention from 1975 onwards. This chronological point is important as there has been a recent tendency to link the emergence of global crime problems with the political collapse of communist states in 1989.

Using the Congresses as a record of the UN's agenda-setting process, the evolution of the content of the agenda can be traced and analysed. Because of the UN's near-universal membership, issues raised as crime problems reflect a wide range of national concerns. In some instances, advocacy of particular problems for criminalisation can produce dilemmas for powerful commercial interests. Referring to the emerging environmental protection regime, Nadelmann commented that, as global regimes develop in these areas, the sanctions levelled against violators can be expected to become increasingly punitive. He further argued that the nature of the violators would 'evolve from the legitimate corporations of today, which are willing and able to contend with civil fines and "white-collar" criminal charges, to entirely criminal organisations and individuals willing to assume greater risks in return for greater profits' (Nadelmann 1990: 523).

Business criminality was raised at the 5th UNCPCTO (Geneva 1975) where there was an examination of changes in the forms and dimensions of criminality which identified both corporate practices (crime in business) and organised crime (crime as business) as capable of corrupting law enforcement and political authority. Thus certain forms of crime were linked not just to the harm that might be done to private or individual security and safety but also harm to the integrity of the state. This perspective was reinforced at the 6th Congress (1980) which looked at crime and abuse of power. It expressed concern about abuses of economic power by both multinational corporations and crime groups as being apparently beyond the reach of the law.

The promulgation of a very broad international crime agenda comes from the 7th Congress at Milan in 1985. This Congress identified 'transnational organised crime' groups as having the capacity to exploit the permeability of national boundaries and carry out multiple illicit operations. The resulting Milan Action Plan had a similar international significance to the, admittedly longer drawn-out, process of the recognition of the imperative to abolish the slave trade. The Action Plan called for the collective endeavour of the international community (Joutsen 1995; Nendik et al. 1995: 88–97) as a response to these problems. Clark viewed the period from 1986 to 1990 as the key period in the raising of the profile of crime issues on the UN's overall agenda (Clark 1995: 26). He cited as examples of this higher profile: the General Assembly's endorsement of the Milan Action Plan (GAR 40/32); the recommendation to ECOSOC by the UN Committee on Crime Prevention of the creation of a global crime prevention and criminal justice network and the UN Secretary-General's 1989 Report reference to concern over crime as generating 'a haunting sense of insecurity' (Clark 1995: 32 citing UN Doc. A/44/1 (1989)).

The 8th Congress (1990) highlighted both a multi-issue suppression item ('organised crime') and a single issue item (terrorism). The Congress considered that both of these required a systematic and co-ordinated response by UN member states. The 1990 Congress was part of the process whereby one form of criminal structure became very visible as a problem which needed to be subjected to a crime-control regime. This is the first time the evolution of international criminal law has been mooted as potentially encompassing a particular form of criminal structure as opposed to specific activities to be criminalised.

This significance was underlined by the fact that the 1990 Congress led to the first ministerial level international crime conference. This was the 1994 World Ministerial Conference on Organised Transnational Crime held, perhaps appropriately, in Naples. The Conference moved the issue on from the recognition stage to the stage of proposals for action with the production of the Naples Political Declaration and Global Action Plan Against Organised International Crime. This document described organised international crime as a 'threat to the security and stability of states'. The influence of the OECD states is evident in the order of the UN's concerns in 1994 as the list prioritises: organised transnational crime, the control of the proceeds of crime and money laundering, crimes already covered by international suppression treaties (drug trafficking and terrorism) and emerging international crime issues (e.g. illegal immigration, illegal traffic in firearms, auto theft and environmental crime). The Declaration may be seen as a reflection of what Hebenton and Spencer (1998) contend is an American-led construction of criminality which, in the post-Cold War era, sees organised crime as 'the new monolithic threat' (cf. Ulrich 1994: 2, citing Senator John Kerry, Dem., Massachusetts). Certainly the theme of transnational criminality was highlighted in President Clinton's address to the UN on the occasion of its 50th Anniversary.

By the late 1990s, the international visibility of the 'white slave' traffic and paedophile crimes put these two crime areas among the leading areas mentioned above (see UN Office for Drug Control and Crime Prevention 'Global Programme against Trafficking in Human Beings', February 1999). The increased visibility of the 'white slave' traffic is partly due to the freer cross-border movements in Europe and evidence of Russian and Eastern European women working in the Western European sex 'industry' (see Savona et al. 1996). The highlighting of paedophile crime can be linked to certain geographical locations being noted for underage sex tourism and the uncovering of networks of organised paedophile activity in the developed states. In this latter case, whether the activity has grown is a matter of conjecture but it is certainly more publicly acknowledged.

A major follow-up to the Naples Political Declaration and Global Action Plan Against Organised Transnational Crime has been the production of a Draft Convention Against Organised Transnational

Crime. Thus the organised crime problem has reached Nadelmann's fourth stage of law creation. But the discussions on the Draft Convention (UN Commission on Crime Prevention and Criminal Justice 1998; see also UN General Assembly 1999) show that organised crime groups have not achieved the status of pirates or slave traders. The concern, rather, is to help states to maximise the use of international co-operation and mutual legal assistance against 'grave manifestations of transnational organised crime'. Examples of these 'grave manifestations' were given as money laundering, trafficking in women and children, and corruption. A particular aim (proposed Article 3) is to persuade all states to have a common offence of 'Participation in a Criminal Organisation', which is inspired by the innovation of US law known as the 'RICO statute'(for a discussion of the development of the RICO – Racketeer Influenced and Corrupt Organizations Act – see Nadelmann 1993).

The Ad Hoc Committee has also been asked by the General Assembly (GAR 53/111 of 9 December 1998) to draw up three additional protocols to the Draft Convention on transnational organised crime. They are to cover the specific offences of the illegal transport and trafficking in migrants; the illicit manufacturing of and trafficking in firearms, their parts and components and ammunition, and trafficking in women and children. These can be seen as areas of private criminality of particular concern in the contemporary period. While organised crime is now clearly an international issue, it must be recognised that its substance is the subject of continuing debate both within law enforcement agencies and legislatures and in academic analyses (see for example Ryan and Rush 1997; the House of Commons Home Affairs Select Committee 1995; US Senate Hearings 1998b; Sénat de Belgique 1998). Alongside the attempt to develop a convention against organised crime, the follow-up work to the Naples Conference (see UN ECOSOC Resolution 1997/22; UN ECOSOC, March 1999, UN Doc. E/CN/1999/3) has also focused on practical law enforcement issues. This is particularly evident in the work of the Senior Experts Group on Transnational Organised Crime and the forty recommendations they agreed in June 1996. For example, Recommendation 3 proposes that states should, 'where feasible, render mutual legal assistance, notwithstanding the absence of dual criminality', and Recommendation 5 proposes that 'direct exchanges of information between law enforcement agencies should be encouraged to the extent permitted by domestic laws or arrangements'.

States are actively pursuing these recommendations, both in developing specific mutual legal assistance treaties (MLATs) and by using the recommendations as part of their broad organised crime control responses. In recent US Senate Hearings (1998a) it was noted that the Senate's ratification of MLATs in 1998 would double the number of those instruments available to the US. The general linkages are also evident in the Preamble to the May 1998 'Pre-accession Pact on Organised Crime between the Member States of the European Union and the Applicant Countries of Central and Eastern Europe and Cyprus' (EU 1998a).

Looking at the treatment of crime at the international level it can be argued that the development of prohibition and suppression regimes has moved on from the rather single issue approach that Nadelmann examined in 1990 to a more system-wide and problem-linked approach. The impetus for this comes from the identification of linkages between drug trafficking, laundering of the proceeds of crime and the recognition of crime as a business with more than *ad hoc* organisational features. It will be seen that this international level change is also evident at the regional level in the response of the European Union.

The European Union

The European Community's formal recognition of crime problems (other than fraud against the Community) commenced in 1975 when the TREVI forum was set up under the intergovernmental Political Co-operation process. This process allowed intergovernmental activity to take place outside the formal framework of the Community treaties and address matters not covered by the treaties. The preoccupation at that time was with domestic and international terrorism, a concern also shared by the wider membership of the Council of Europe which developed a regional Convention on Terrorism in 1977 (see further Anderson et al. 1995).

The first systematic examination of private criminality occurred in 1985 as the member states examined the Community-wide aspects of drugs and arms trafficking and cross-border movements of stolen goods. This was carried out by TREVI Working Group III. Further consideration of the Single Market Programme, with its requirement of free movement for people, goods, services and capital (as set out in the Single European Act of 1986) involved EC members in what was to become a more continuous engagement with the problems of transnational private criminality. Other crime problems soon recognised as of common concern were fraud and money laundering. Because of the closed nature of the TREVI forum the Community did not really set out a crime-control agenda in public until the early

1990s when the Treaty on European Union with its Justice and Home Affairs 'pillar' was negotiated. This process was accompanied by an associated institutional development, the Convention establishing the European Union Police Office (Europol). This agenda-setting process was continued by the 1997 Treaty of Amsterdam (see Anderson et al. 1995; Gregory 1998).

The Europol Convention explicitly refers to serious organised crime as the rationale for Europol working with the police and other law enforcement agencies in member states. However, that involvement can relate to any one or combination of 26 crime categories including drug trafficking, illegal immigrant smuggling, auto theft, money laundering and paedophile crime. With the advent of this agency, the EU became more capable of helping member states to discharge their obligations under international criminal law conventions, such as the 1988 Vienna Convention on Drug Trafficking and regional agreements such as the Council of Europe Money-laundering Convention. It could also aid in developing the processes of transnational policing through mutual legal assistance. Within the EU area, in addition to the Pre-accession Pact on Organised Crime (EU 1998a), intergovernmental means were further developed to tackle organised crime in advance of the more protracted route of the negotiations on an International Convention against Organised Crime. The March 1998 Justice and Home Affairs Council 'Joint Action', for example, made it a criminal offence to participate in a criminal organisation in the Member States of the EU (EU 1998b; and see also EU 1998c). In addition, the Baltic Sea States group (EU members, accession countries and Russia) began operating a task force on organised crime in the Baltic Sea region in 1996. The general agreement between the governments in this instance has been based upon the pragmatic foundation of exploiting the limits of national legislation.

Although some aspects of these multinational efforts at controlling private criminality can be criticised as the 'shopping list' approach (Joutsen 1995: 299) or mere ritual exercises (Williams and Savona 1995), there is evidence of organised crime, such as drug trafficking and money laundering, prompting a defined and multidimensional response which will, in totality, amount to a transnational prohibition and suppression regime.

Control of corruption

It can also be argued that the response is actually moving beyond the creation of standard prohibition and suppression regimes and improving the policing co-operation processes of extradition and mutual legal assistance. There is a recognition that the problem of criminals being apparently beyond the reach of the law needs to be tackled by developing a regime to control crime facilitation through corruption (see van Duyne 1997; Brademas and Heimann 1998; Bray 1998). This is evidence of international concern with the effects of private criminality on the actual practice of policing in states. The Interpol Director of Legal Affairs, Souheil El Zein, has commented that 'Corruption is an important aspect of organised crime – it is often the cornerstone of the activities of some criminal organisations – the officials who have been corrupted are frequently those who should have been investigating the criminal activities, or at least contributing to such investigations' (El Zein 1998: 29).

During 1996 the UN General Assembly called for 'Action Against Corruption' and adopted an 'International Code of Conduct for Public Officials'. In so doing the General Assembly expressed the view that it was

> *Concerned* at the seriousness of problems posed by corruption, which may endanger the stability of societies, undermine the values of democracy and morality and jeopardise social, economic and political development. *Also concerned* about the links between corruption and other forms of crime, in particular organised crime, including money laundering.
>
> (UN General Assembly Resolution GAR 51/59)

In the same month GAR 51/191 of 16 December 1997 contained a 'Declaration Against Corruption and Bribery in International Commercial Transactions' and invited member states 'to take appropriate measures and co-operate at all levels to combat corruption and bribery in international commercial transactions' (UN General Assembly Resolution GAR 51/59).

The Declaration required Member States

1   To take effective and concrete action to combat all forms of corruption, bribery and related illicit practices in international commercial transactions;
2   To criminalise such bribery of foreign public officials.

By 1999 the UN response to the problem was encapsulated in a 'Global Programme against Corruption: An Outline for Actions' (UN Office for Drug Control and Crime Prevention 1999a). This 'outline for action' referred to corruption 'as a major problem in society and noted 'the increasing involvement of organised crime on extortion and corruption' (pp. 6–7).

Since 1994 the OECD began focusing on point two above, through the recommendations (OECD 1997) which ask member countries to 'criminalise the bribery of foreign public officials in an effective and co-ordinated manner by submitting proposals to their legislative bodies by 1 April 1998'. At the regional level, since 1994, the Council of Europe has been discussing a framework convention to define common principles in the fight against corruption and a criminal law convention against corruption. By 1996 the Council of Europe's Committee of Ministers had adopted an Action Plan against corruption and in 1997 the conference of Ministers of Justice recognised, by Resolution 1 of their 21st Conference, the link between corruption and organised crime. By 1998 the Council of Europe had moved two significant stages in its anti-corruption strategy. Firstly, it had ready a Draft Criminal Law Convention on corruption. This Convention was signed by Member States on 27 January 1999. Secondly, the Committee of Ministers adopted, in May 1998, R(98)7 which authorised the adoption of the Partial and Enlarged Agreement and established a monitoring group of states (GRECO). Aigrot describes this as 'the first international mechanism to monitor compliance with international commitments in the field of corruption' (Aigrot 1998: 25). The Council of Europe has also joined with the Commission of the European Community in the 'Octopus Project' which aims to help 16 European states in political and economic transition tackle corruption and organised crime.

Having reviewed the historical evolution of the international concern regarding criminal actions for private gain, the analysis will now examine the visibility of that agenda in the proposals for an International Criminal Court (ICC). It will be argued that a measure of the seriousness with which states are prepared to treat the international effects of serious private criminality would be the presence or absence of offences such as drug trafficking in the remit of an ICC.

Proposals for an International Criminal Court[1]

It might be argued that the idea of an international criminal court is a clear expression of a less Hobbesian view of international relations. Such a court could be seen as consistent with a notion of global security, where individuals as well as states have obligations related to international norms of behaviour, expressed in legal form. An international criminal court is also linked to states' accepting modifications upon their national prerogatives regarding jurisdiction and political sovereignty. However, the history of recent efforts to set up such a court reflect a reluctance on the part of some states (significantly the USA) who have resisted the development of a supra-national jurisdiction. This contrasts with their evident support for the development of international criminal law mechanism, suppression treaties, etc, to support municipal criminal law jurisdiction.

The first initiative for such a court came in 1937 when a League of Nations conference proposed a 'Convention for the Prevention and Punishment of Terrorism and for the Creation of an International Criminal Court' (ICC) (Gianaris 1991: 93). There was renewed interest in this idea after World War II following the war crimes trials. However, it was not until 1989 that the UN General Assembly requested the International Law Commission (ILC) to address the issues associated with an ICC. In 1990 and 1991 the General Assembly further requested the ILC to consider questions of international criminal jurisdiction. Finally, in 1992 and 1993 the General Assembly requested the ILC to draft a Statute for an ICC. The ILC prepared the Draft Statute by 1994 and it was reviewed by an *ad hoc* committee, set up by the General Assembly. In the 1994 session of the ILC the hope was expressed that a narrow but significant list of 'hard to challenge' crimes could be included in the remit of the ICC. Among these, as well as war crimes, were: aggression, international terrorism and drug trafficking. However, the ILC, in the 1995 session, could only actually agree upon the inclusion of aggression, genocide, war crimes and serious violations of human rights. The General Assembly then established a Preparatory Conference in 1995 to draw up a Convention to establish the ICC and this was produced in April 1998.

The ILC Report and Draft Statute (UN International Law Commission 1993) was based upon the ILC's work on a 'Draft Code of Crimes against the Peace and Security of Mankind' which was first produced in 1991. The proposed Court's jurisdiction was defined, firstly, in Article 22 as covering genocide (Genocide Convention 1948), grave breaches of the 1949 Geneva Conventions regarding the treatment of wounded and sick military personnel on active services and the 1949 Geneva Conventions on the Treatment of Prisoners of War. Article 22 also gave the Court jurisdiction over unlawful seizures of aircraft (1970 Convention), crimes against civil aviation safety (1971 Convention), apartheid and related crimes (1973 Convention), crimes against internationally protected persons (1973 Convention), hostage-taking (1979 Convention) and crimes against maritime safety (1988 Convention).

The emerging nature of the treatment of private criminality in international criminal law and the problem of achieving consensus on the bases for international action, were reflected in the more circumscribed consideration of the extension of the court's jurisdiction to other crimes. Under Article 26(b) it was proposed that a specific State, or States (either where a crime was committed or where a suspect is held) might give the Court jurisdiction in respect of:

> 2(b) crimes under national law, such as drug-related crimes, which give effect to provisions of a multilateral treaty, such as the 1988 United Nations Convention against Illicit Traffic in Narcotic Drugs and Psychotropic Substances, aimed at the suppression of such crimes and which having regard to the terms of the treaty constitutes exceptionally serious crimes.

The commentary provides a very useful way for the non-legal specialist to appreciate the current treatment of individuals as 'criminal' in international law. At present only the crimes listed under Article 22 constitute 'international crimes'. The Article 26(b) crimes come under the scope of 'treaties which merely provide for the suppression of undesirable conduct constituting crimes under national law' (pp. 279–81).

As discussions progressed, the 1996 Draft Code was reduced in its crime coverage by the exclusion of threat of aggression, colonial domination, mercenaries and illicit drug trafficking. The 1996 draft Code only covered, formally, five crimes: aggression, genocide, crimes against humanity, crimes against UN and associated personnel and war crimes. But the actual articles did also cover apartheid (Article 18(f)), institutional discrimination as a crime against humanity and environmental damage (Article 20(g)) as a war crime. Ambos noted that international terrorism was not included because of imprecise definition as an offence category and drug trafficking was excluded as ILC members did not consider this as a crime against the peace and security of mankind (Ambos 1996: 534).

McCormack and Simpson (1994) identified some important cautionary points that need stating before the stage of the adoption of the ICC statute is considered. They reminded interested parties that there are at least three different and not very compatible ways of defining criminality in international law: illegal acts by states, state acts giving rise to individual responsibility, and proposals that some individual acts be dealt with under international law. Additionally, Ambos made the realist point that 'the more punishable conducts included in the jurisdiction of an international court, the fewer the states that will be willing to accept the jurisdiction' (Ambos 1996: 523). Using the ILC work on the Draft International Criminal Code and the Draft Statute for an ICC, it is *very* evident that there was only a consensus within the ILC on a restricted international crime agenda. The consensus, from within this body of legal experts, was clearly only in favour of listing crimes against the peace and security of mankind and crimes against humanity and thus it did not encompass private criminality as discussed here. Moreover there was evidence that, as Ambos suggested, states confronting national political interests at the pre-signing stage were more likely to sign a 'narrow' rather than a 'broad' statute for an ICC. The 99-article draft statute was reported as having 1,700 'brackets', i.e. areas of disagreement. An example of national sensitivities was provided by US concerns over the ability of the Court to try US military personnel. It was reported that Jesse Helms, Republican chairman of the Senate Foreign Relations Committee, maintained that any treaty that failed to give Washington veto power would be 'dead on arrival' when sent for ratification (*The Times* 30 March 1998; see also UN Law Report (33) 1998: 30–1).

The UN General Assembly invited member states to a Diplomatic Conference to establish the ICC in 1997. This was held in Rome in July 1998 and the 'Rome Statute of the International Criminal Court' was agreed on that occasion (UN 1998a; UN 1998c). One hundred and sixty states took part and the Chair of the Drafting Committee was M. Cherif Bassiouni of Egypt, a keen advocate of the ICC concept. At this conference, States agreed upon a restricted form of ICC. Firstly, it was to have jurisdiction only where national courts cannot or will not act (Article 17). The only crimes over which the Court will have authority were listed as: genocide, crimes against humanity and war crimes. It might gain jurisdiction over 'aggression' if a separate set of negotiations can eventually agree a justiciable definition. The limited nature of the ICC's potential jurisdiction is well illustrated by Article 7 'Crimes against humanity'. Under Article 7.1(g) 'enforced prostitution' is such a crime, but Article 7.1 also states that this is only a crime against humanity if 'committed as part of a widespread or systematic attack directed against any civilian population' (UN 1998c:1004–5), a considerable limitation. The possibility of other crimes coming within the Rome Statute was never formally considered. Indeed only one state, even informally, raised such a possibility. The reasons for this were set out in Annex I E to the Rome Statute. In this the Diplomatic Conference recognised that terrorist acts, by whomever and wherever perpetrated and whatever their forms, methods or motives, are crimes of concern to the international community that international trafficking of illicit drugs is a very serious crime, sometimes destabilising the political and social economic order in states

and was

> *Deeply alarmed* at the persistence of these scourges, which pose serious threats to international peace and security *Regretting* that no generally acceptable definition of the crimes of terrorism and drug crimes could be agreed upon for inclusion, within the jurisdiction of the Court.

The Conference therefore invited a future Review Conference with reference to Article 123 of the Rome Statute to 'consider the crimes of terrorism and drug crimes with a view to arriving at an acceptable definition for their inclusion in the list of crimes within the jurisdiction of the Court'. Thus one form of private criminality may come within the jurisdiction of the ICC but, clearly, not for some years. Such internationally acknowledged private crimes therefore remain, in terms of international response, at the level of international suppression treaties which set minimum requirements for municipal criminal law and inter-state law enforcement co-operation.

Behind this vaunted success of the Rome Conference, characterised by Robin Cook, the British Foreign Secretary, as 'a strong court with wide powers' (*Weekly Hansard*, 20 July 1998, col. 803), there were some significant problems. Firstly, because of fears of proceedings against US military personnel overseas the United States did *not* append its signature and neither did China. Secondly, achieving the 60 ratifications necessary to give effect to the Statute is likely to be a lengthy process. Additionally, the ICC is expected, in operation, to work within the parameters of the principle of 'complementarity'. That is to say, its jurisdiction is only to be exercised when a state is unable to fulfil its international obligations by reason of the collapse of its criminal justice system through war or internal conflict.

If finally established and operational, the ICC would create a new form of transnational police work through the ICC's independent prosecutor. The provision will allow this office to initiate investigations and prosecutions under its own power. States would be expected to enable their police forces to work on behalf of the prosecutor. But, as pointed out above, this police work would be confined to war crimes or crimes against humanity.

Conclusions

This chapter has used the literature on international criminal law and built on Nadelmann's important contribution to identify the growing scope of international concern and response over certain forms of private criminality and to see whether any criminal actions other than piracy or slave trading are deemed so indefensible as to render the perpetrators the common enemy of mankind. The answer to the latter question, it was argued, might be found in any extension of the International Criminal Court's jurisdiction beyond war crimes and crimes against humanity. This has not yet happened. However, the list of private criminal actions regarded as of international concern has increased and the organised form of criminality, and the corrupting power of criminal groups, have been recognised as additional causes for concern.

States, in viewing crime as an element in their new and expanded definition of security, have responded by emphasising the development of well established modes of co-operation such as extradition and mutual legal assistance, supplemented by additional 'suppression' treaties, such as the 1988 Vienna Convention on Drug Trafficking, the Council of Europe Money Laundering Convention, the proposed Organised Crime Convention and the efforts to control corruption. All of these serve three broad purposes: firstly, to establish a particular offence or offences in all municipal law systems; secondly, to require states to prosecute or extradite in such cases; and, thirdly, to encourage all relevant forms of law enforcement co-operation. With regard to the fulfilling of the latter purpose, generally speaking states have not sought to create any form of supranational policing. This is a point reflected in an article in Interpol's 75th Anniversary book where the comment was made that 'there is still no real life agent from Interpol', there is only the liaison officer seconded from, and working with, national police forces (Kendall 1998: 306). Similarly, the EU has created, by a public international law convention, the European Union Police Office (Europol) as an aid to criminal intelligence data collection, exchange and analysis in support of nationally based investigations.

This is perhaps not surprising as there has been no move to change the fundamental principle of international law that a state can only exercise criminal law policing and jurisdiction within its own territory, overseas possessions or with respect to its own registered ships and aircraft outside territorial limits. Examples of 'judicial imperialism' exist but remain few in number. Moreover, practices which might at first glance appear to be precursor examples of transnational policing activities in the nineteenth century (against pirates and the slave trade) in fact, relied upon the tasking of the navies of a small number of states using the 'sovereignty-free' space of the high seas. It has also been established, from the historical examples, that even all that international effort was only partly successful in crime prevention and control. In the contemporary period, it is even more clear that the drug trafficking suppression regime is facing a very resilient illicit commodity traffic.

What has been established, however, is that national criminal justice systems – in their activities of investigation, apprehension and prosecution – have been increasingly drawn into working with, and in support of, other national criminal justice systems within frameworks established by international criminal law treaties and regional or international action programmes. Private criminality, at least in certain forms, is no longer an exclusively national matter and thus there is clearly a transnational dimension to national policing, but this is transnational policing which operates within an evolving inter-state consensus, not through supra-national means.

Note

1 The author would like to acknowledge the help of Steven Neff, Edinburgh School of Law, who commented on an earlier draft of this chapter.

References

Aigrot, L. (1998) 'Experiences of the Council of Europe', *Europe 2000*, 18 September, pp. 23–35.

Ambos, K. (1996) 'Establishing an International Criminal Court and International Criminal Code', *European Journal of International Law*, Vol. 67, pp. 519–44.

Anderson, J. (1997) 'Economic Implications of Piracy, 1750–1850', in D. Starkey, E. S. van Eyck van Heslinga and J. A. De Moor (eds), *Pirates and Privateers*, Exeter: University of Exeter Press.

Anderson, J. B. (1991) 'An International Criminal Court: An Emerging Idea', *Nova Law Review*, Vol. 15, pp. 2–3.

Anderson, M., den Boer, M., Cullen, P., Gilmore, W., Raab, C. and Walker, N. (1995) *Policing the European Union: Theory, Law and Practice*, Oxford: Clarendon Press.

130   *Frank Gregory*

Arlacchi, P. (1998) 'The Strategic Role of International Organisations in Fighting Drug Trafficking', pp. 39–41 in R. Kendall (ed.), *Interpol: 75 Years of International Police Co-operation*, London: Kensington Publishers.

Bassiouni, M. (1974) 'An Appraisal of the Growth and Developing Trends of International Criminal Law', reprinted in J. Dugard and C. van den Wyngaert (eds) (1996), *International Criminal Law and Procedure*, Aldershot: Dartmouth.

Bassiouni, M. and Blakesley, C. (1992) 'The Need for an International Criminal Court in the New World Order', *Vanderbilt Journal of Transnational Law*, Vol. 25, No. 2, pp. 157–82.

Brademas, J. and Heimann, F. (1998) 'Tackling International Corruption', *Foreign Affairs*, Vol. 77, No. 5, pp. 17–22.

Bray, J. (1998) 'Companies, Corruption and Competition', *The World Today*, August/September, pp. 223–35.

Chalk, P. (1998) 'Low Intensity Conflict in South East Asia: Piracy, Drug Trafficking and Political Terrorism', *Conflict Studies*, No. 305/306, London: Research Institute for the Study of Conflict and Terrorism.

Chatterjee, S. K. (1980) *Legal Aspects of International Drug Control*, Dordrecht: M. Nijhoff.

Clark, R. S. (1995) *The United Nations Crime Prevention and Criminal Justice Programme*, Philadelphia: University of Pennsylvania Press.

Cockcroft, L. (1998) 'Causes and Consequences of the End of Toleration of Grand Corruption', *Europe 2000*, 18 September, pp. 16–22.

Crawford, J. (1996) 'Proposals for an International Criminal Court', in J. Dugard and C. van den Wyngaert (eds), *International Criminal Law and Procedure*, Aldershot: Dartmouth.

Dugard, J. and van den Wyngaert, C. (eds) (1996) *International Criminal Law and Procedure*, Aldershot: Dartmouth.

van Duyne, P. (1997) 'Organised Crime, Corruption and Power', *Crime, Law and Social Change*, Vol. 26, pp. 201–38.

El Zein, S. (Director, Legal Affairs, Interpol General Secretariat) (1998) 'The Role of ICPO-Interpol in International Police Co-operation', in R. Kendall (ed.), *Interpol: 75 Years of International Police Co-operation*, London: Kensington Publishers.

European Union (1998a) 'Pre-accession Pact on Organised Crime between the Member States of the European Union and the Applicant Countries of Central and Eastern Europe and Cyprus', 28 May 1998, http://www.ue.eu.int/jai/article.asp?lang=en&id=69808331.

European Union (1998b) 'Progress Report on Organised Crime to the Cardiff European Council', 6 August 1998 http://www.ue.eu.int/jai/article.asp?lang=en&id=79807303.

European Union (1998c) 'Joint Action on Making it a Criminal Offence to Participate in a Criminal Organised Action', 21 December 1998, http://www.ue.eu.int/jai/article.asp?lang=en&id=39807586.

Galeotti, M. (1993) 'Perestroika Perestrelka, Pereborka; Policing Russia in a Time of Change', *Europe–Asia Studies*, Vol. 45, No. 5, pp. 769–86.

Gianaris, W. N. (1991) 'The New World Order and the Need for an International Criminal Court', *Fordham International Law Journal*, Vol. 16, No. 1, pp. 59–76.

Gregg, R. W. (1964) 'The UN and the Opium Problem', *European Journal of Political Research*, Vol. 26, pp. 82–601.

Gregory, F. (1995) 'National Police Forces in International Services', pp. 1260–8 in J. Lovenduski and J. Stranyer (eds), *Contemporary Political Studies 1995*, Belfast: Political Science Association.

Gregory, F. (1996) 'The United Nations Provision of Policing Services (CIVPOL) within the Framework of "Peacekeeping" Operations: An Analysis of the Issues', *Policing and Society*, Vol. 6, pp. 145–61.

Gregory, F. (1998) 'Policing Transition in Europe: The Role of EUROPOL and the Problem of Organised Crime', *Innovation*, Vol. 11, No. 3, pp. 287–305.

Hebenton, B. and Spencer, J. (1998) 'Law Enforcement in Societies in Transition', *European Journal of Crime, Criminal Law and Criminal Justice*, Vol. 6, No. 1, pp. 29–40.

House of Commons (1995) Select Committee on Home Affairs Report *Organised Crime* (HC 18-I), London: HMSO.

Joutsen, M. (1995) 'The Emergence of United Nations Criminal Policy: The Fourth Session of the United Nations Commission on Crime Prevention and Criminal Justice', *European Journal of Crime, Criminal Law and Criminal Justice*, Vol. 3, No. 3, 351–76.

Kendall, R. (ed.) (1998) *Interpol: 75 Years of International Police Co-operation*, London: Kensington Publishers.

Lloyd, C. (1968) *The Navy and the Slave Trade*, London: Frank Cass.

Lubbock, B. (1993) *Corsairs, Cruisers and Slavers*, Glasgow: Brown and Co.

McCormack, K. and Simpson, B. (1994) 'The International Law Commission Draft Code of Crimes against the Peace Security of Mankind', in J. Dugard and C. van den Wyngaert (eds), *International Criminal Law and Procedure*, Aldershot: Dartmouth.

McDonald, W. F. (ed.) (1997) *Crime and Law Enforcement in the Global Village*, Cincinnati, OH: Anderson Publisher Co.

Malenczuk, P. (1997) *Akehurst's Modern Introduction to International Law*, 7th revised edition, London: Routledge.

Marquand, P. (1995) 'Law without Borders: The Constitutionality of an ICC', *Columbia Journal of Transnational Law*, Vol. 34, No. 1, pp. 73–148.

Meneffe, P. (1990) 'Piracy, Terrorism and the Insurgent Passenger', in N. Ronzitti (ed.), *Maritime Terrorism and International Law*, Dordrecht: M. Nijhoff.

Murray, D. (1997) 'Chinese Pirate Communities, 1750–1850', in D. Starkey, E. S. Van Eyck van Heslinga and J. A. De Moor (eds), *Pirates and Privateers*, Exeter: University of Exeter Press.

Nadelmann, E. (1990) 'Global Prohibition Regimes: The Evolution of Norms in International Society', *International Organization*, Vol. 44, No. 4, pp. 479–526.

132   *Frank Gregory*

Nadelmann, E. (1993) *Cops across Borders: The Internationalization of US Criminal Law Enforcement*, University Park PA: Pennsylvania State University Press.

Nendik, K., Zyharz-Shaw, S. and Lovell, B. (1995) 'The World Ministerial Conference on Organised Transnational Crime – Background, Results and Follow-up', *European Journal of Crime, Criminal Law and Criminal Justice*, Vol. 3, No. 1, pp. 88–98.

OECD (1997) Council Revised Recommendations C97/123/Final on Combatting Bribery in International Business Transactions, 23 May 1997, *International Legal Materials*, Vol. 36, p. 1016.

Pugh, M. (ed.) (1994) *Maritime Security and Peacekeeping*, Manchester: Manchester University Press.

Ronzitti, N. (ed.) (1990) *Maritime Terrorism and International Law*, London: M. Nijhoff.

Rubin, A. P. (1997) *The Law of Piracy* (2nd edn), New York: Transnational Publications Inc.

Ryan, F. and Rush, G. (eds) (1997) *Understanding Organised Crime in Global Perspective*, London: Sage.

Savona, E. U., di Nicola, A. and da Col, G. (1996) 'Dynamics of Migration and Crime in Europe: New Patterns of an Old Nexus', *Transcrime: Working Paper*, No. 6.

Schwarzenberger, G. (1950) 'The Problem of an International Criminal Law', reprinted in J. Dugard and C. van den Wyngaert (eds) (1996), *International Criminal Law and Procedure*, Aldershot: Dartmouth.

Sénat de Belgique (1988) 'Commission parlementaire chargée d'enquêter sur la Criminalité Organisée en Belgigue – Rapport final fait par MM. Coveliers et Dermedt', Document 1 326/9, session 1998–9, 8 December 1998.

Slaughter, A. M., Tulumello, A. S. and Wood, S. (1998) 'International Law and International Relations Theory: A New Generation of Interdisciplinary Scholarship', *American Journal of International Law*, Vol. 92, pp. 367–97.

Starkey, D., van Eyck van Heslinga, E. S. and De Moor, J. A. (eds) (1997) *Pirates and Privateers*, Exeter: University of Exeter Press.

Thomas, H. (1997) *The Slave Trade*, London: Picador.

Ulrich, C. (1994) 'The Price of Freedom: The Criminal Threat in Russia, Eastern Europe and the Baltic Region', *Conflict Studies*, No. 275, London: Research Institute for the Study of Conflict and Terrorism.

United Nations (1998a) Diplomatic Conference of Plenipotentiaries on the Establishment of an International Criminal Court (Rome Statute) Final Act, UN Doc. A/CONF, 183/10, 17 July 1998.

United Nations (1998b) International Convention for the Suppression of Terrorist Bombings, 9 January 1998, *International Legal Materials* (1998), Vol 36, p. 249.

United Nations (1998c) Rome Statute of the International Criminal Court, UN Doc. A/CONF 183/9, 17 July 1998, *International Legal Materials* (1998), Vol. 37, pp. 999–1111.

United Nations Commission on Crime Prevention and Criminal Justice (1988) Chairman's Report of the Working Group on The Naples Political Declaration and Global Action Plan against Organised Trans-national Crime. UK Foreign and Commonwealth Office, May 1998.

United Nations Economic and Social Council (ECOSOC) (1988) Convention Against Illicit Traffic in Narcotics Drugs and Psychotropic Substances (Vienna Convention), 19 December 1988, E/CONF. 82/15.

United Nations Economic and Social Council (ECOSOC) Resolution 1997/22, 'Follow-up to the Naples Political Declaration and Global Action Plan against Organised Transnational Crime,' 21 July 1997.

United Nations Economic and Social Council (ECOSOC) (1999) 'Strategies for Crime Prevention: Discussion Paper on the theme of the Eighth Session of the Commission on Crime Prevention and Criminal Justice', Report of the Secretary-General, UN Doc. E/CN.15/1999/3, Vienna: UN Commission on Crime Prevention and Criminal Justice, March 1999.

United Nations General Assembly Resolution GAR 51/59 (1996) on Action Against Corruption, 12 December 1996, *International Legal Materials* (1997) Vol. 36, p. 1039.

United Nations General Assembly Resolution GAR 51/191 (1996) containing UN Declaration Against Corruption and Bribery in International Commercial Transactions, 16 December 1996, *International Legal Materials* (1997) Vol. 36, p. 1043.

United Nations General Assembly (1999) 'Report of the Ad Hoc Committee on the Elaboration of a Convention against Transnational Organised Crime on its third session, held in Vienna from 28 April to 3 May 1999', UN Doc. A/AC.254/14; V.99–84210(E), Vienna: May 1999.

United Nations International Drug Control Programme (UNDCP) (1997) *World Drug Report*, Oxford: Oxford University Press.

United Nations International Law Commission (1993) 'Report of the Working Group on a Draft Statute for an International Criminal Court', 16 July 1993, *International Legal Materials* (1994), Vol 33, p. 253.

United Nations Office for Drug Control and Crime Prevention (1999a) 'Global Programme against Corruption: An Outline for Action,' UN. Doc. V–99–80875(E), Vienna: February 1999.

United Nations Office for Drug Control and Crime Prevention (1999b) 'Global Programme against Trafficking in Human Beings: An Outline for Action', Vienna: February 1999.

United States Senate (1998a) Hearing before the Committee on Foreign Relations, 'Extradition, National Legal Assistance, and Prisoner Transfer Treaties', 105 Congress, 2nd Session, 15 September 1998, S. Hrg. 105–730, Washington DC: US Government Printing Office, 1998.

United States Senate (1998b) Hearing before the Select Committee on Intelligence, 'Current and Projected National Security Threats to the United States', 105 Congress, 2nd Session, 28 January 1998, S. Hrg. 105–587, Washington DC: US Government Printing Office, 1998.

Vagg, J. (1995) 'Rough Seas – Contemporary Piracy in South East Asia', *British Journal of Criminology*, Vol. 35, No. 1, pp. 63–80.

Williams, P. and Savona, E. U. (eds) (1995) 'The UN and Transnational Organised Crime', *Transnational Organised Crime*, Special Issue, Vol. 1, No. 3.

Zmeeski, A. and Tarabin, V. (1996) 'Terrorism: The Need for Co-ordinated Efforts by the World Community', *International Affairs*, Vol. 42, pp. 83–9, Moscow.

5 Policing the virtual launderette

Money laundering and global governance[1]

James Sheptycki

Introduction

Money laundering, seen as the *sine qua non* of organised crime in the contemporary period, was an unspoken concept for criminologists in the middle years of the twentieth century. Donald Cressey, one of the most ardent pursuers of organised crime in the academic discipline, did not use the term. He was, however, well acquainted with its practice. He described in functional terms the role of the 'money mover', a person or group of persons whose role is first to hide the source of illegally obtained money and second to facilitate its re-introduction into the banking system so that it can be put to work just like any other form of capital (Cressey 1969: 234). Mary McIntosh noted, twenty-five years ago, that legitimate enterprises were a necessary part of the racketeer's business concerns. Legitimate business 'fronts' provide a way by which extortionate transactions can be disguised among a regular flow of uniform payments and she mentioned the provision of laundry services *first* among the examples of types of business enterprise that can be used, not only as a cover for criminal activity, but also as a conduit through which money from the clandestine economy can be moved into the regions of the 'upper world' (McIntosh 1975: 51). According to William Gilmore (1993) the term 'money laundering' entered popular usage during the 1970s, around the time of the Watergate scandal. Michael Sindona, the Vatican Banker involved in the so-called Banco Ambrosiano affair of the mid-1980s, was able to define the term succinctly as 'switching dirty money to clean money' (quoted in Reid 1996: 207). Given the historical connection with the laundry business noted by McIntosh, and the function of moving criminal money so as to disguise its criminal origins described by Cressey, it is perhaps not surprising that the term 'money laundering' has come to be a part of the criminological lexicon.

Estimating the amount of 'dirty money' in the economy is fraught with difficulty, but such estimates that can be derived are invariably impressive. Thus, for example, a special issue of the *Annals of the American Academy of Political and Social Science* contained estimates for the USA of between US $12 and $18 billion annually in 1933 rising to about $55 billion in 1963, figures which were seen as 'almost fantastic' (Tyler 1963: 105–7). Estimates of the amount of illicit capital flowing in the veins of the global financial system ranged between $300 and $500 billion annually in the mid-1990s (Gilmore 1995: 25; Quirk 1996). These figures are large indeed, but criminologists and economists working in this area agree that there is, in fact, no way to quantify the precise extent of the clandestine economy. This is not least because of the interpenetration of the licit and illicit finance. It is, for instance, a commonly held view that the Mafia in Italy derives more income from its 'legitimate' business interests than from its criminal activities (Nelken 1997). Further, research has shown an increasing overlap between organised crime, corporate crime and ordinary business (Passas and Nelken 1993). Some criminologists even maintain that organised crime is simply another form of capitalist enterprise, dissolving the distinction between 'dirty' and 'clean' money altogether (Ruggerio 1996), but a thorough reading of McIntosh's earlier work (1975) can inoculate the novice against this extreme view. At the very least, since economic relations in clandestine markets cannot make use of the law of contract, organised crime ultimately depends on extreme forms of violence in order to enforce and maintain business ties and agreements. As McIntosh notes, organised crime 'depends on the violence that some of their number are willing to carry out or to threaten. This violence is controlled and purposeful' (p. 56). At a fundamental level, it is the use of extreme violence that helps distinguish what we mean when we use the term 'organised crime'. For this reason, if for no other, the boundary between illicit and licit capital is a concern for policy-makers thinking about transnational organised crime. But the topic raises other extremely interesting questions for those interested in the further evolution of transnational policing and of the global state-system.

The purpose of this chapter is twofold. The first aim is to outline the forms that money laundering has taken and the development of national and international control measures that have been undertaken thus far. The survey of control measures will look at initial developments in the USA, on the Financial Action Task Force (FATF), money-laundering policy in the European Community and selected developments in western Europe. In order to shed further light on the practices of transnational policing in this area, some examples of police investigations in this field will also be considered. This will provide something of a measure not only of the law as it is written, but also as it is practised. The goal is to illuminate the control choices available to, and created by, policy-makers and the dilemmas that arise from them. The second aim is to look at new forms of 'electronic money' (Weatherford 1997). This is important since electronic money is said to entail problems of control; because electronic money is in cyberspace, which is everywhere and nowhere, simultaneously (or very nearly) in bank accounts in Switzerland, Grand Cayman, Jersey and around the corner at the local shopping mall, it has been argued that territorially based governments will find it increasingly difficult to control or direct its flows. Hence the claim to the 'hollowing out of the state' (Bottoms and Wiles 1995, 1997) and even a suggestion that the state has become 'impotent' (Castells 1997). Concomitantly it is often argued that the difficulty in tracing money further blurs the distinctions that officials, at both national and transnational levels and in both state and non-state institutions, are able to make between legitimate and illegitimate financial dealings. This line of argument goes on to suggest that surveillance is consequently necessary for all banking-type transactions (UNDCP 1998). Examining the policing of economic transactions and banking practices offers the interested observer a window onto the emergent practices of global governance. This analysis focuses on questions about *how* governance works in the transnational context, and only tangentially considers *why* such changes in governance have come about (cf. Miller and Rose 1990).

Money laundering techniques

There is one sense in which organised crime and capitalist enterprise are congruent; both are practices intended to generate profit. The essence of such enterprise is that capital be re-invested in future economic activity. However, criminal entrepreneurs attract the efforts of formally designated agents of social control, that is: police agencies of various types. There are a variety of avenues that policing may take to control criminal enterprise, but the juncture at which raw cash is introduced into the banking system has come to be seen as a point of particular vulnerability. While minor offenders can 'spend as they go', more successful criminal entrepreneurs may amass cash in quantities so large that it is very difficult to safe-guard or spend unobtrusively. There is a story that is often told in police circles, possibly apocryphal, which relates to a cache of cash amassed by Pablo Escobar, of the

Medellín cartel in the late 1980s. It is said that Escobar had at that time some $400 million in currency hidden in a house in Los Angeles that he could not ship across the border to Mexico. Eventually, the basement flooded and the money became waterlogged and rotted away (Arrasia 1996: 228, citing an article in the *Los Angeles Times*, 26 June 1991). Thus, there is a need for professional money manipulators – people whose job it is to move the cash into and through the banking system. There are many techniques that can be used to achieve this, but they all have the same basic aims: to conceal the true ownership and origin of the money, to maintain control of that money, and move it within the banking system in order to take maximum advantage of it.

Money laundering has three stages: placement, layering and integration (extending the 'laundering' metaphor we could say: wash, spin and dry). At the placement stage, cash deposits enter the financial system for the first time. This is not as easy as it might seem, since in many advanced capitalist countries there are formal requirements that banks verify the identity of their clients and report large cash transactions including deposits and the opening of accounts – a threshold figure of US $10,000 being a typical figure. By concentrating on deposit takers, that is on the 'placement stage', the first step in an audit trail can be established by investigators. One tactic for getting around this requirement is that of 'smurfing', whereby the services of numerous individuals of innocuous appearance are employed to make large numbers of small transactions (always under the $10,000 threshold). This facilitates the injection of large quantities of cash into the banking system without triggering the reporting system. Non-bank financial institutions, such as casinos, cheque-cashing services and *bureaux de change* are well suited to cash placement using this method. Authorities in the Netherlands have reported some success with prevention measures which regulate more closely the business of *bureaux de change* (Ministry of Justice 1992), this is reportedly less easy to do with casinos (UNDCP 1998). Another tactic used to avoid compulsory reporting rules is to ship cash to banking jurisdictions which do not have such regulations, with the concomitant risk of discovery as the money is physically transported across international boundaries. Many jurisdictions have followed the lead of the United States and passed legislation which allows for the interdiction and seizure of cross-border cash shipments that are derived from serious criminal enterprise (especially drug trafficking), these countries include the G7 nations and numerous others such as Australia, Ireland and the Netherlands. In 1992 US Customs authorities reported 862 seizures of outbound cash shipments totalling $42 million in value (Gilmore 1995: 42). In the United Kingdom, the Criminal Justice (International Co-operation) Act 1990 was introduced which, in part, enabled police and customs officials to seize cash being brought into or out of the UK where there is reason to believe that it could be the proceeds of drug trafficking (Drage 1993: 61–2).[2]

The third way that illicit capital can be banked and moved is within 'underground' or traditional banking systems which bypass the regulatory authorities who oversee transactions that occur in the formally established financial sector. According to Grabosky and Smith (1998), these systems are centuries old and are part of the market infrastructure of Middle-eastern and Asian business. Typically, under such arrangements a person wishing to transfer money would deposit it with a 'banker' – most likely an ordinary merchant – and, in return, would be given a distinctive 'chit' or 'chop' redeemable at another specified location, very often the business premises of a relative or close associate of the 'banker'. Thus, a person could deposit a sum of money, say US $100,000, with a merchant in San Francisco, travel to Hong Kong and receive the cash equivalent (less an agreed commission) in Hong Kong dollars upon presentation of the receipt. It is important to recognise that these traditional banking systems are indigenous to traders across North Africa, throughout the Middle East and South-east Asia, China and the Far East and they enable a considerable amount of global money movement. Estimates range anywhere between US $100 and $300 billion passing through these transnational banking networks per annum (Grabosky and Smith 1998: 178). While these underground banking systems facilitate a sizeable amount of global cash flow (which, with electronic mail and other new forms of communication, may be growing), this is dwarfed by the estimated $175 billion a *day* of international monetary transactions (Nelken 1997: 269).

Once criminal proceeds have been 'placed' in the financial system, the next stage is that of 'layering'. This involves the creation of a long list of transactions, across many jurisdictions and between many shell companies, creating complex layers of financial contrivance. This creates an audit trail that is extremely difficult to follow, even for the most practised forensic accountant. There are three principal techniques used in the process of layering. The foremost is the simple use of international wire transfers. As mentioned above, there is a considerable amount of money moved around in the global banking system, only a small portion of which is connected with actual trade or investment decisions, the remainder is 'hot capital' looking for short-term speculative investments in liquid or semi-liquid possession (Arlacchi 1993). Within this vast flow of money it is possible to lose the identification details of sender and beneficiaries. In the mid-1990s the US government, through the Federal Financial Institutions Examination Council (FFIEC), moved to require all 27,435 domestically chartered banks, thrift institutions and credit unions to register the name, address and account number of the person (that is, the non-financial institution originator) who initiated a given payment order as well as corresponding details pertinent to the beneficiaries of the transaction (Greenberg 1994: 59–60).[3] Similar measures in the global banking system or at the regional level are correspondingly difficult to engineer, partly because of the incremental complexities that arise in a much bigger system and also because the system's regulators are not part of a coherent institutional framework (UNDCP 1998). Even in the European Union where there is a modicum of bank law harmonisation, differences in national financial surveillance systems do not facilitate the degree of co-ordinated information sharing possible within the United States (Thony 1996; Pieth 1998). However, the USA has tried to influence developments at the transnational level. It has asserted a seigneurial invitation, through such varied organs as the OECD, the IMF and the G7, to create a global anti-money-laundering regime. This process will be examined in more detail below.

Trade in various forms of financial instrument, such as securities, currency or commodity deals or collateral for loans, also offers opportunities to lengthen the paper trail. This is a second tactic that can be used to confound investigators, which has the additional, and attractive, possibility of being profitable if the trading is sharp.[4] Lastly, layering makes use of offshore companies in jurisdictions with strict banking secrecy laws. Shell companies act as depositories for cash, make loans for businesses owned by the self-same individuals who are seeking to cleanse the 'dirty money', or to send double invoices to businesses thereby confusing the audit trail (Drage 1993: 60–1). The offshore banking system is central to the internationalisation of money transfer, estimates made in the mid-1990s suggested that there was approximately £400 billion in the UK offshore banking sector (Jersey, Guernsey and the Isle of Man) (Bamber 1998) and some US $500 billion in the Cayman islands (UNDCP 1998: 28). A government report on UK offshore centres (referred to as the Edwards Report, after its author Andrew Edwards, a former Whitehall civil servant) was published in November of 1998 (*The Economist*, 28 November 1998). Edwards revealed that bank deposits in Jersey grew from an estimated

£7.9 billion in 1980 to nearly £100 billion by 1997. Further, the report estimated that around one third of the wealth of the world's 'high net worth individuals' was held in the offshore banking system, inferring that a substantial proportion of offshore wealth was held there for the purposes of tax avoidance. The Channel Islands' share of that global market was estimated to be only 5 per cent. The islands were, however, said to be 'in the top division of offshore centres', and 'judicial and prosecution systems, regulation, and co-operation with other jurisdictions are remarkably good'. While the islands were praised 'for giving exemplary assistance in many cases of drug trafficking, fraud, tax offences and money laundering', the report also acknowledged that 'the extent of disreputable business is hard to judge', and that the scale of tax evasion and fraud 'unusually hazardous' to guess.

Thus we arrive at the 'integration' stage, which is the last step in the process. After moving through multiple transactions in the banking system, the laundered funds eventually emerge in investment portfolios which appear no less clean than any other. Such investments may take the form of unit trusts, single premium life insurance, or other forms of securities, and even the acquisition of already established legitimate business enterprise. Obviously, the management of these potentially vast portfolios requires the services of professional accountants and lawyers – some of these persons will be aware of the particular taint that a given investment portfolio carries, others need not be, further complicating the paper trail.

American measures against money laundering

Criminal enterprise has had to engage with the banking sector for as long as there have been clandestine markets. Having said that, attempts to police this interface are relatively recent. Measures against money laundering first arose in the context of the 'war on drugs' in the USA (Grabosky and Smith 1998: 176). According to Ethan Nadelmann, American legislative efforts to confront this newly defined criminal practice began with the Bank Secrecy Act of 1970, but the legal requirements that banks report cash transactions that exceeded $10,000, or that individuals transporting more than $5,000 in cash out of the USA submit currency reports, were not effectively enforced until the mid-1980s (Nadelmann 1993: 388).[5] These laws created three new types of record, the Currency Transaction Report (CTR), pertaining to banking transactions over the $10,000 mark and the Currency or Monetary Instruments Report (CMIR), pertaining to expatriation of money over the $5,000 level. Additionally, there was the Foreign Bank Accounts Report (FBAR); a reporting requirement for any US citizen with a foreign bank account with an amount exceeding $1,000. It is probably safe to say that it was not until the mid-1980s that a sufficient archive of such records, and the technical and administrative expertise necessary to exploit them, had been built up to enable systematic enforcement to be pursued on the basis of these auditing mechanisms. In 1984 US law enforcement sources were able to report that multi-agency task forces, comprised of US Assistant Attorneys and agents from the Internal Revenue Service (IRS), Customs, the Federal Bureau of Investigation (FBI), the Drugs Enforcement Agency (DEA) and the Board of Alcohol, Tobacco and Firearms (ATF), had been operating with some success and that computerised data analysis of these banking records had been used to discover 'unusual patterns of money movements through the banking system' (OCDE Task Force 1984: 62). Efforts in this domain of policing were new, and the processes involved were described as 'highly sophisticated, technical and time-consuming', but despite the difficulties, teams of investigators in a number of locations were 'working to mine this lode' of data (p. 62). It was explained that the 'financial approach' provided an innovative way to detect persons involved in the drug trade, 'traffickers often make illegal currency transactions . . . [for example, they] fail to pay their full share of income tax' (p. 61). This was seen as an additional point of vulnerability. Thus the goal was 'to make full use of financial investigative techniques, including tax law enforcement and forfeiture actions, in order to identify and convict high-level traffickers and to enable the government to seize assets and profits derived from high-level drug trafficking' (p. 61).

However, these techniques also led to 'the discovery of financial irregularities that do not relate to drug transactions' (p. 63). It became something of a mantra for agents working in this field that all 'high-level' drug dealers were, by definition, engaged in financial irregularities, but that all persons engaged in financial irregularities were not drug traffickers. Peter J. Quirk, an advisor to the IMF's Monetary and Exchange Affairs Department, noted in 1996 that the forms of monitoring for tax evasion and for money laundering focus on individuals and economic entities and their revenues and are thus quite similar. According to him, improving both tax collection and anti-laundering systems could be expected to yield increased results because laundered income from crime is most often the subject of tax evasion. He further argued that the need for an efficient monitoring system was widely agreed, even by those generally averse to more than minimal taxation, because it allowed for the reduction of assessed rates of taxation generally (Quirk 1996). Others argued, in the UK context, that high visibility prosecutions for facilitating tax evasion were needed to force professional compliance from tax advisors and others who offer financial services to clients who may be involved in serious criminal activity (Bridges 1996). The extension of the money-laundering law to tax evasion would, it was argued, make it more difficult for professional advisors to provide services and remain immune from prosecution for money laundering and related offences. At the same time, it was also argued that extending monitoring into the area of tax evasion would make it easier for investigating authorities to prove an offence of criminal conspiracy involving financial advisors who might handle, even unknowingly, the proceeds of crime. Various types of criminal enterprise could be mentioned here, pension funds skimmers and other types of fraudster, for example, but there are non-criminal reasons for making use of the offshore banking sector. Individuals might have reason to secrete their wealth in the context of divorce proceedings so as to avoid the financial consequences of litigation, or as a device for controlling the portioning of familial inheritance. In other cases medical practitioners seeking to avoid pre-emptively the predations of pernicious lawyers who pursue malpractice claims (which may or may not be legitimate), may also seek refuge in the offshore banking system. Others might seek to secrete their wealth simply to avoid (or evade) paying tax.

The distinction between tax avoidance and tax evasion is not obvious. There are perfectly legal ways to avoid paying taxes. For example, *The Economist* reported that in the four years to 30 June 1998, Rupert Murdoch's News Corporation and its subsidiaries paid US $238 million in corporate taxes world-wide. In the same period its consolidated pre-tax profits were almost US $4 billion, an effective tax rate of around 6 per cent. Basic corporate tax rates in the USA, Australia, and the UK, the principal countries in which Murdoch's companies do business, are 35, 36 and 30 per cent respectively. By comparison, Disney, a US-based global media empire, paid about 31 per cent in corporate tax over the same period. News Corporation is able to avoid paying taxes by funnelling funds through offshore shell companies in some 60 financial havens. For example, News Publishers, incorporated in Bermuda (a tax haven), made around £1.6 billion in the seven years to June 1996 (*The Economist*, 20 March 1999). Tax avoidance, the exploitation of loopholes which can arise through drafting errors and linguistic ambiguities in income tax laws, is entirely legal. Simple evasion, not paying taxes on otherwise taxable income, is illegal. There is a fine line between evasion and avoidance; sometimes that line is merely the difference between having competent and incompetent legal advice. Certainly the latter is cruder and need not draw on the expertise of tax lawyers and accountants; it is to the tax specialist what stuffing a mattress full of cash is to bankers.

In short, there are many fish in the financial sea besides money launderers who might have reason to desire secrecy, not all of whom are on the wrong side of the criminal law. Thus, as Grabosky and Smith (1998) point out, 'any system of monitoring commercial transactions would be seen as a gross violation of privacy'. Further, 'even the most law abiding citizens would be disinclined to leave an electronic trail of all their financial transactions' and 'few would welcome a financial system becoming an instrument of surveillance' (p. 181). However, that is precisely what has been engineered. There was reportedly a debate among members of the various investigative task forces operating across the USA when this surveillance infrastructure was in its infancy about the propriety of investigating these non-drug related cases. It was suggested that 'fishing expeditions' – that is, simply targeting any individuals who come to light as a result of this system of surveillance – were to be eschewed in preference for 'proactively targeting' individuals and organisations involved in the drug trade. However, these surveillance practices, and the concomitant evolution of the legal practices that underwrite them, proceeded apace. According to some legal analysts, during the 1990s prosecutors developed an avid interest in 'white-collar' cases. Armed with weapons conceived to combat narcotics and organised crime, prosecutors turned towards white-collar cases as well, and not without success. Thus tax fraud and other similar cases came to be commonly converted into harsher RICO Act and money-laundering cases, with their accompanying asset forfeiture features. 'Incremental drift' or 'mission creep' is one way to characterise this development. It might also be postulated that, having created the legal means to control organised crime's money-laundering practices, the Trojan Horse was positioned in the bank. Once there, access and control over many other forms of tainted money was possible, not least of which was money due to the Internal Revenue Service. Be it 'mission creep' or 'Trojan Horse', the outcome has been that those convicted of these types of white-collar offences are now being subjected to harsher punitive sentences even as civil forfeiture provides a new way to punish offenders (Morvillo and Bohrer 1995).[6]

The capacity of this emerging financial policing surveillance infrastructure is great, the income generated for law enforcement no less so. In the mid-1990s it was observed that, by using asset forfeiture laws,

US federal law enforcement generated revenue for itself that was in excess of $500 million annually. Further, local and state law enforcement had accrued a similar figure nationally (Payne 1999: 30). In 1997 the US Federal government estimated that it would seize about $1.5 billion from bank accounts in New York, Florida, Texas and California over the course of the coming two years. The Treasury Department's Financial Crimes Enforcement Network (FinCen) was co-ordinating a multi-agency initiative which included local and state police in those four jurisdictions in co-operation with the DEA, FBI, IRS and US Customs. At the heart of this enterprise was a national financial database with software capable of determining links between seemingly unconnected businesses and bank accounts. According to one FinCen official 'the database is so sophisticated that in five minutes or less it can produce a profile of a person's financial history, business contacts, employer, assets, real estate titles, even a list of neighbors who can be contacted by investigators. That information can be fed into another database that establishes a "daisy chain" of individuals, businesses and bank accounts linked with the original suspect' (LEN, No. 467, 1997). There was some legal wrangling during the middle part of the decade as the Supreme Court wrestled with the issue of whether or not asset forfeiture amounted either to an 'excessive fine' (in violation of the Eighth Amendment to the US Constitution, which states: 'Excessive bail shall not be required, nor excessive fines imposed, nor cruel and unusual punishments inflicted'), or to 'double jeopardy' (the Fifth Amendment to the Constitution, which states in part: 'No person shall . . . be subject for the same offence to be twice put in jeopardy . . . nor shall private property be taken for public use without just compensation'). With regard to the objections under the Eighth Amendment, the government argued, successfully, that such seizures were primarily remedial in nature, intended to permit the removal of tools of the drug trade. With regard to the arguments under the Fifth Amendment, the Supreme Court ruled, in a majority decision, that civil forfeiture was not a punishment, but rather served non-punitive goals, such as encouraging property owners to make sure their property was not used for illegal purposes (LEN 1993; LEN 1996b).[7] There were attempts to curb these powers through legislation. In 1993 Henry Hyde (Rep. Illinois), introduced a bill that would have put basic limitations on asset forfeiture which, according to him, would ensure that innocent people were not penalised. He argued that 80 per cent of the people whose property was seized under the Comprehensive Drug Abuse Prevention and Control Act of 1970 were never even charged, much less convicted of a crime. The limitation he sought on asset forfeiture was simply that, in order for an application to take control of financial assets to be upheld, the individual concerned would have to be successfully prosecuted for a drug-related crime. Since the standard of proof in civil forfeiture is lower than it is in criminal proceedings this would have been a significant break on forfeiture takings. Hyde's and other's efforts have, to date, been fruitless.

Improvements in surveillance capacity continued apace and, at the end of the decade, the controls on the movement of money out of the USA were tightened even further. 'Using computers like radar', records of banking transactions could be scanned for patterns of financial transactions that were 'thought to be consistent with money laundering' (LEN 1996a). In 1997 new Treasury Department guidelines followed the successful Operation Eldorado in the New York area, where the threshold for external wire transfers out of the United States was lowered to $750, initially on an experimental basis. This experiment was undertaken after it had been observed that, to account for the estimated $1.3 billion sent to Colombia from New York City annually, the 25,000 Colombian families living there would have to be repatriating approximately $50,000 per year each; but the median annual household income for this group was only $27,000 (LEN 1997a; IELR 1997a). This new and much lower threshold was aimed at the estimated 1,600 outlets providing financial services; street-corner cheque-cashing services and major non-bank money transmitters (for example Western Union and American Express). It required them to register the identity (including providing photographic records) of any individual sending more than $750 abroad to particular countries (Colombia and the Dominican Republic) and, further, imposed a duty to report any suspicious activity, such as multiple transactions just under the $750 level.[8] These are called Geographic Targeting Orders (GTOs). GTOs were established on the basis of a previously little-used statutory provision which enabled the Secretary of the Treasury to require special reporting and record-keeping by financial institutions in specific geographic areas where necessary to fulfil the purposes of the Bank Secrecy Act. A representative of the Non-Bank Fund Transmitters Group (an industry association representing Western Union, Thomas Cook, American Express and other similar corporations) estimated that this would increase the filings of these institutions 'by a million pieces of paper a year' (LEN 1997c), a heavy burden on the industry. The extension of financial transaction surveillance of this type was justified by the suggestion that these measures had forced criminal entrepreneurs to resort to shipping raw cash. It was claimed that the result was an increasing number of seizures of cash shipments by Customs. In one instance so credited, US Customs officials found more than $10 million stuffed into stereo systems destined for Colombia (LEN 1996a).

Surveillance over the money-moving system acted, in substantial part, by making counter staff in banks and other financial institutions responsible for enhanced record-keeping. Such 'responsibilisation' (cf. Garland 1996, 1997; Sheptycki 1998b) made them primary agents of surveillance, enhancing governmental knowledge of money movement necessary to the functioning of the electronic financial surveillance system. We can characterise this responsibilisation strategy as 'governance at a distance' (Garland 1999), since employees in the private sector have been given a key role in a governmental strategy. However, the core task has remained the province of state agents and significant financial rewards return to these agencies as a result of these efforts through the mechanism of asset forfeiture law.

Bilateral and multilateral action on money laundering

Interventions against 'dirty money' were based initially on unilateral action by sovereign states, primarily the USA. According to Ethan Nadelmann (1993: 315), US prosecutors, police agents, and courts had resorted to unilateral, extra-territorial means of collecting evidence from abroad in these kinds of cases, and thus the principal incentive for many foreign governments to negotiate MLATs with the United States was the desire to curtail such action by American authorities. Although Nadelmann referred to mutual legal assistance treaties intended to facilitate evidence-gathering generally, it seems quite clear that these motivations were partly, even considerably, animated in the context of the emergent anti-money-laundering regime. Since the principal targets of extra-territorial evidence-gathering in money-laundering cases have been multinational banks and other corporations (some based in the USA, some in other jurisdictions), which had, in the past, been persuaded to perform tasks allotted by US governmental authorities by threat of court orders, anti-trust actions and export controls against US affiliates (as well as direct actions against individuals in positions of responsibility in these institutions), there was a strong incentive to negotiate a legal basis for such evidential requests.[9] Indeed, since banks outside the USA had been compelled in a number of instances to hand over to American law enforcement authorities financial documents stored in branches outside the United States, often counter to financial secrecy laws and other blocking statutes, there was felt to be a need to normalise these procedures under law.

An early example of this process was the negotiation of an MLAT between the USA and Switzerland which was ratified in both countries in 1977 after almost a decade of negotiations. This MLAT concerned several matters, many to do with 'translation' between the terminology of US and Swiss law so as to facilitate meaningful communications. However, a significant priority for the Americans was to persuade the Swiss government to lower the veil of secrecy laws that ensured confidentiality within their banking system. Given this goal, the Justice Department could not but be dismayed when the Swiss government created a Federal Act on International Mutual Assistance in Criminal Matters (IMAC) in 1981 which codified the provisions of the MLAT that had been signed four years previously. Dismayed because of provisions contained in two Articles, one which required that 'upon receipt of a request for assistance, the requested State shall notify . . . any person from whom a statement or testimony or documents, records, or articles of evidence are sought' (Swiss MLAT, Article 36(a), quoted in Nadelmann 1993: 335). The direct consequence of such a provision would be to warn any suspect of the fact that they were under investigation, allowing them time to shift funds away from the gaze of investigators. The other provision that US authorities found irksome was the requirement that requests for assistance include both 'the subject matter and nature of the investigation of proceeding' and 'a description of the essential acts alleged or sought to be ascertained' (Article 29(1)(a), quoted in ibid., p. 335) thereby notifying any suspect under investigation precisely how the case against them was being pursued and, perhaps, lumbering prosecutors with an untested theory vulnerable to being undermined through questioning in Swiss courts. In the late 1990s the Swiss government remained committed to the general principles of banking secrecy but, in the face of arguments that Switzerland had not gone far enough in developing an anti-money-laundering surveillance capacity, also argued that, in fact, Swiss bank secrecy law was weaker than the professional secrecy afforded to doctors, lawyers and Ministers of State. On balance, it seems that, with regard to the proceeds of crime, banking secrecy in Switzerland has been rolled back substantially (IELR 1996: 254; IELR 1997b: 6) and this is a consequence of the Swiss government's participation in the multilateral efforts of the Financial Action Task Force (FATF), about which more below.

Since the negotiation of the MLAT between the USA and Switzerland there have been a number of developments: the 1988 UN Convention against Illicit Traffic in Narcotic Drugs and Psychotropic Substances asked for comprehensive criminalisation of money laundering as well as the expansion of instruments for the confiscation of the proceeds of crime; the 1989 Basle Statement of Principles on Money Laundering laid the groundwork for outlawing anonymous accounts; and a host of MLATs (that facilitate the tracing, freezing and forfeiture of funds), too numerous to mention, are the most salient examples. According to Mark Pieth, Professor of Jurisprudence at the University of Basle, Switzerland, 'this process is certainly remarkable and we all know of the decisive role the US have played in initiating it' but 'the changes would not have come about so quickly and so radically if the other major developed countries had not readily cooperated' (1998: 160). Indeed, the Commonwealth Scheme for Mutual Assistance in Criminal Matters, endorsed at a meeting of Commonwealth law ministers in Harare in 1986 was seen as a step ahead of the USA in developing a truly transnational response for the control of criminal enterprises (Nadelmann 1993: 386). The Commonwealth Scheme drew on the UK Drug Trafficking Offences Act (1986) which brought into UK law provisions for confiscation of the proceeds of drug trafficking. This scheme dealt with three matters (McClean 1988: 187–8); the first were tools for identifying, locating and assessing the value of property believed to be the proceeds of criminal activity. The second dealt with the seizure and forfeiture of such proceeds and the third dealt with various procedures for securing foreign forfeiture orders.

The first binding multilateral agreement to contain measures against money laundering was the United Nations Convention Against Illicit Traffic in Narcotic Drugs and Psychotropic Substances (1988), sometimes known as the Vienna Convention (Gilmore 1991). This Convention addressed both the criminalisation of money laundering and the confiscation of criminal proceeds as well as a host of other enforcement concerns, such as interdiction at sea, the use of 'controlled delivery', and other 'proactive' policing techniques. With regard to confiscation, the Convention explicitly stated that a requested party could not decline to act in the tracing, identification, seizure, freezing and forfeiture of criminal proceeds on the grounds of bank secrecy. It ensured that signatory states would treat drug-related money laundering as a serious criminal offence, thereby creating a transnational law enforcement regime. Significantly, it contained no preventative measures *per se*, rather, the somewhat elliptical philosophy of the Convention was taken from the 1987 UN Conference on Drug Abuse and Illicit Trafficking, to wit that 'it is necessary to ensure vigorous enforcement of the law in order to reduce the illicit availability of drugs, deter drug related crime, and contribute to drug abuse prevention by creating an environment favourable to efforts for reducing illicit supply and demand' (quoted in Gilmore 1991: 1). Thus, the thinking behind this international co-operation regime appears to be general deterrence of illicit drug activity through vigorous law enforcement activity among the bank books. The principles of the Vienna Convention have been resoundingly echoed in subsequent agreements. For example, the Council of Europe Convention on Laundering, Search, Seizure and Confiscation of the Proceeds of Crime – which was the first international instrument to extend the crime of money laundering beyond drug-related scenarios to include the proceeds of all 'serious crime' – also focused on the use of the criminal law in the pursuit of general deterrence through the threat of asset seizure and, failing deterrence, to make the crime pay the costs of its own criminal law enforcement.

To be sure, enforcement was not the only modality. A contrast to the focus on criminal law enforcement can be found in the Basle Statement of Principles on Money Laundering. This statement took as its starting point the vested interests the banks have in maintaining a positive image. The tactics propounded in the Basle Statement were *prudential* in nature, focusing on the sagacity of banks scrutinising the financial components held within their minimum capital requirements. The aim was for banks to protect themselves from the negative consequences that 'grey' or 'dirty' money might have for their capital reserves by establishing a system of minimum standards for the quality of assets held in investment portfolios. It was thought that the interests of the banks could best be protected by prudential limits which restrict their exposure to illicit capital, or to borrowers who might perpetrate fraud. By undertaking such prudential measures, banks and other financial institutions have sought to minimise the disruptive potential that illicit capital might bring with it. Not accidentally, these efforts also serve to maintain perceptions of the trustworthiness and sound sobriety of the banks among investors and depositors alike.

The Financial Action Task Force (FATF), mentioned earlier, is a free-standing specialist body concerned with the multilateral enhancement of anti-money-laundering capacity. It was established by the G7 nations in July of 1989 and its membership extends to 26 countries representing the advanced capitalist economies.[10] The FATF was *ad hoc*, nested in the OECD Headquarters in Paris, with a budget of some 4 million French francs and a staff of three (Gilmore 1995, 1999). It was not created as a permanent international organisation and its mandate has had to be extended, once in 1991 and a second time in 1994 for five years. In the annual report for 1998 a five-year plan for the years 1999–2004 was agreed (IELR 1998). Its mandate has been to assess the regime for international co-operation against money laundering, connected with all forms of 'serious crime' and it has done so through a series of 'mutual evaluations' between and within each signatory's banking system. FATF documents do not expressly define what is meant by the term 'serious crime'. This vague term clearly extends system surveillance beyond the single-minded pursuit of drug money. Recommendations put forward by the FATF suggest that 'the laundering of drug money is frequently associated with the laundering of other criminal proceeds. Given the difficulty of bringing evidence of drug money laundering specifically, an extension of the scope of this offence, for instance to the most serious offences, such as arms trafficking, etc., might facilitate prosecution' (Sherman 1993: 22). The FATF recommended further that the offence of money laundering be extended to 'all offences that generate a significant amount of proceeds' (p. 23). In 1990 the FATF set forth 40 recommendations intended to set the stage for a comprehensive anti-money-laundering strategy and this has been the bench-mark for the mutual evaluations. Three core measures were regarded as constituting the general thrust of the specific proposals, those being: (1) that each member state should ratify and implement the 1988 Vienna Convention; (2) that financial secrecy laws should be conceived so as not to inhibit money-laundering investigations; and (3) to increase multilateral co-operation and mutual legal assistance in such investigations and prosecutions and that bars on extradition in money-laundering cases should be minimised (Gilmore 1995: 101). In the 1998 annual report, the FAFT noted that 'the most notable trend is the continuing increase in the use of money launderers of non-bank financial institutions and of non-financial businesses relative to banking institutions [sic]' (IELR 1998: 309). This phenomenon is well known to criminologists and is a characteristic of deterrence tactics generally; the term used to describe it is 'displacement'. In this instance the anti-laundering regime was displacing the crime of money laundering from one institution (banks) to others. As a result, the deterrence practices of the anti-laundering regime had to expand into these other institutions, for example helping the offshore insurance industry which was thought to be particularly vulnerable (IELR 1998: 315).[11]

Be that as it may, the FATF itself has been chiefly concerned to nurture the systematic monitoring of the banking process in order that illicit funds come to light. Its 40 recommendations do not constitute a binding legal agreement or treaty, but rather constitute a general framework for co-operation. The FATF practises 'governance at a distance', a strategy which depends partly on procedures of self-assessment and mutual evaluation and it was frequently claimed that the threat of peer-group review (backed up by the possibility of blacklisting for non-compliance) was the best catalyst to action. This 'soft law' approach has been seen as necessary, since member states require flexibility so that the eccentricities of national legal systems, financial systems and other local factors can be taken into account. The FATF recommendations were an attempt to set out a strategy by which the component institutions of the financial system could become responsible for combating money laundering. This responsibilisation, or self-policing, strategy aims to involve all actors in the international financial system in targeting 'dirty money', without (it is hoped) operating as a drag on legitimate transactions. This strategy has been pursued with both member states and non-member states in the pursuit of a global anti-money-laundering regime. The FATF was concerned to oversee the implementation of these various recommendations and with examining cases of money laundering that come to light in order to gauge changing trends and keep banking practice sharp.

A key development in the European context over the course of the 1990s was the development of Financial Intelligence Units (FIUs). According to Thony, FIUs were created in response to a European Directive issued on 10 June 1991 which established the obligation to report suspicious financial operations (Thony 1996: 258). Financial Intelligence Units amass information from the financial sector, collate it (sometimes with reference to other forms of criminal intelligence) and disseminate it among a network of similar institutions. Thony usefully classified FIUs under three types, those being: police, judicial or administrative 'options'. An example of the police-centred model is that found in the UK, where the Economic Crime Unit within the National Criminal Intelligence Service (NCIS) has 'the function of centralizing and filtering reports of suspicions' (p. 265). Because bankers may be reluctant to report mere suspicions to an agency whose responsibility it is to create evidence for criminal prosecutions, with the attendant possibility of wrongly ensnaring their clients in a criminal investigation, 'only countries, such as the United Kingdom, with a high level of confidence in the police authorities can expect results from this option' (p. 267). The judicial option can be found in Denmark, Switzerland, Iceland and Luxembourg and 'because of the guarantees of independence that it offers, the judicial option probably inspires greater confidence in financial circles than the police option' (p. 268). The FinCen structure in the USA, discussed earlier, epitomises the administrative model, but France has also opted for a roughly similar approach with the establishment of La Traitement du Renseignement et Action contre les Circuits Financiers Clandestins (TRACFIN). This is 'unquestionably the one [model] that provides the best interface between the banking and financial world and the investigative and prosecuting authorities' (p. 270) but one of the many drawbacks Thony cites is that bankers 'do not want to become agents of the internal revenue authority' and 'are sometimes reluctant to pass on information to a service that reports to the same supervisory authority as the tax collection services' (p. 271). Detailed analysis of the many FIUs in existence shows that the idiosyncrasies of each national FIU tended to belie the simplicity implied by Thony's typology. Indeed, the creation of the Unusual Transactions Reporting Office (MOT) in the Netherlands, which introduced an independent agency with responsibility for centralising information pertinent to money-laundering investigations while preventing 'unjustified intrusions into private life and to safeguard the interests of financial institutions', shows the limitations of the typology (p. 275).

One consequence of this variety of institutional forms, according to Thony, is that 'isolation [within host states] is an inherent feature of FIUs . . . [and] this isolation naturally prompts the services to seek cooperation with a view to data exchange, even when they are not assigned that role by law' (p. 275). Bilateral agreements between FIUs facilitate this form of data exchange, but the main difficulty has concerned the confidential nature of the information. As Thony noted 'in the absence of legislative harmonization, the current variety of FIU legal structures may be an obstacle to the effective development of cooperation' (ibid.). The Egmont Group, which first came together in June 1995, is a forum wherein FIUs around Europe can share this information. The Egmont Group meets with regularity but has no formal status either in national or international law (pp. 275, 279) and little is, as yet, known about the functioning of this institution. It might be accurate to characterise it as a prototype for a transnational superstructure for co-ordinating information exchange emanating from the surveillance of financial transactions records. A measure of the enormity of this task is suggested by noting that legislation brought into being in the UK in 1993 (an amendment of the Criminal Justice Act), which rendered the failure to report suspicious transactions a punishable offence, created a flood of reports to the National Criminal Intelligence Service (NCIS). In the absence of clear guidelines as to the criteria for assessing what constitutes 'suspiciousness', the NCIS received in excess of 15,000 reports in 1994. A subsequent information campaign calculated to ensure a degree of restraint and judgement resulted in a slight drop and the NCIS received only 13,700 reports in

1995. In the Netherlands, the MOT received some 23,000 reports in 1994 (pp. 265–6, 272). The sheer number of reports raises questions about the ability to make systematic use of them and the suggestion that successful counter-measures against money-laundering operations may be the result of the more or less random successes of 'data mining'.

The fight against drug trafficking and money laundering, Thony notes, 'increasingly resembles a combat campaign, and intelligence is one of the weapons of war' (1996: 274). The war footing has resulted in some problematic features of the emerging global anti-money laundering regime. Grabosky and Smith noted that the FATF recommendations included the creation of a global currency tracking system and sanctioned the use of covert or 'sting' operations (1998: 180). Only a few people writing in this area have observed that the use of these intrusive methods, what police call 'proactive investigations', raise problems of accountability as well as posing significant ethical, political and legal questions (Marx 1988; Fijnaut and Marx 1995). These techniques have been accorded some considerable recognition of success by the law enforcement community, but operational utility is not the only measure. The next section explores the *modus operandi* of police in these cases.

'The sting' in anti-money-laundering operations

On 22 October 1995, US President William J. Clinton used the occasion of his 14-minute speech before the 50th Anniversary of the UN to propound initiatives against international organised crime – especially narcotics trafficking and money laundering. Other leaders speaking at previous UN anniversary occasions had focused on more traditional areas of the United Nations' concerns: war and peace, poverty, hunger and education. Clinton's speech was considered by some to be aimed at the domestic US audience (IELR 1995a: 493), the speech took aim at 'international organised crime' in order 'to promote the safety of the world's citizens'. This seems an unambiguous signal to a variety of players in the international system of a continuing shift in US foreign policy. Only one year previously, the Centre for Strategic and International Studies in Washington DC brought together 'leaders of the financial, intelligence and law enforcement communities' to discuss global organised crime which was characterised as the new 'Empire of Evil' (Raine and Cilluffo 1994). With respect to the US national perspective, one contributor to the conference (Buck Revell, formerly the FBI's principal deputy for criminal investigations, counter-terrorism and counter-intelligence activities) argued for wholesale sharing of intelligence within and between US law enforcement and intelligence agencies and recommended the establishment of a national criminal information centre which would enable the US federal government to strategically manage the response to organised crime. With specific regard to money laundering, Stanley E. Morris, Director of the Financial Crimes Enforcement Network (FinCen), advocated more training and technical assistance to further enable direct on-line sharing of information between the various agencies in the law enforcement enterprise (both in the US and abroad). He also urged the enhancement of co-operation and information sharing with the private sector, especially banks and other financial institutions. Morris was particularly concerned that the USA work to raise standards in the financial sector around the globe and he advocated training programmes for overseas bank personnel so that they could participate in the system's surveillance. A summation by James Woolsley, the then director of the CIA, conceptualised global organised crime as a 'threat to international security' suggesting, since some weaker governments would be unable to withstand these security risks, that there was therefore a need for the 'global community' to develop legal mechanisms.

Clearly US policy regarding the functioning of the international system in its broadest sense has a significant crime control element to it and it is likely the seigneurial rights that accrue to the dominant state power will shape the nature of that system. So how have these crime-control policies been enacted on the world stage? There are a number of examples of successful police undercover operations, but one of the most notable was Operation Dinero which came to fruition in 1995. This operation began in 1991 when US and UK authorities co-operated in mounting a long-term undercover operation in Anguilla, a British colony not far off the coast of Puerto Rico. Anguilla is largely economically dependent on the production of tropical fruits and fishing, but its bank secrecy laws made it a minor offshore banking centre, bringing in welcome hard currency to the island. Notwithstanding its status as a British colony, Anguilla is just the sort of 'weak state' US officials meant when they put forward the idea that international organised crime is capable of corrupting governments, thus creating the need for protection by the 'international community'. There seems an obvious geopolitical logic in targeting money laundering in an offshore centre so close to the US mainland.

The undercover operation basically consisted of establishing an elaborate 'sting' set up with funds from the DEA. Using 12 'front' companies and 51 bank accounts to provide currency exchanges, cashiers' cheques, holding companies, wire transfers, help setting up shell corporations and the whole panoply of miscellaneous services that are required in the international banking sector, the undercover operatives actively sought out business from suspect money launderers and associates. Over the course of its three-year operation the bank was reported to have carried out 92 cash transactions valued at US $39.5 million and 291 non-cash transactions totalling US $8.9 million. A further US $4.3 million was seized from money couriers in the final phase. The bank itself was a 'virtual' entity, existing only as an electronic address and on stationery. The operation was first constituted by US and UK police in co-operation with the Attorney-General of Anguilla, but came to involve police agencies in other countries, notably Italy, Spain, and Canada. Only the Anguillan Attorney-General knew that one of the class B banks on the island was an undercover operation run by the DEA and the IRS Criminal Investigative Division. As the investigation progressed, money was traced through the global banking system to Spain, Gibraltar, Cyprus, Canada, Italy, and the United States, as well as Latin America. Writing in the *International Enforcement Law Reporter*, Bruce Zagaris noted that 'the detective work conducted by the police in both Europe and North America, including their ability to continue the operation over a three year period and the level of penetration by law enforcement officials, demonstrates success. The operation's success has shown law enforcement officials in several countries the utility of undercover operations. It is likely to be repeated in the future in that officials will establish not only undercover sting banks, but also other financial institutions, such as broker-dealer firms, mutual fund operations, and exempt insurance companies to lure and trap money launderers' (IELR 1995b: 41).

Not all such undercover operations go so smoothly. Passas and Groskin (1995) have pointed out that undercover operations can stumble into political minefields in which political actors may be affected by, or seek to manipulate, the outcome of such police operations to further their own ends (see also Brodeur, this volume). 'This is very shaky ground', they suggest 'and most law enforcement agencies do not have the requisite knowledge or expertise to assess such nuances from a distance' (p. 305). While co-operation between UK and US authorities in the Operation Dinero case did not seem to involve such problems, there are other examples of 'sting' operations where results were not entirely positive. The ramifications of transnational police operations in the international domain can be far-reaching indeed. One such example is that of Operation Casablanca which eventually escalated into a full-scale diplomatic altercation between Mexico and the United States. The extent of the diplomatic tension was evident in exchanges between the Senate majority leader Trent Lott and Reyes Heroles, the Mexican Ambassador to the United States. The former stated bluntly in a letter to President Zedillo that Operation Casablanca 'is not "inadmissible" or a "violation" of your sovereignty. It is a decisive action against ruthless criminals'. Mr Heroles replied that the undercover operation was 'an act of a criminal nature similar to the crimes it was supposed to uncover' (*New York Times*, 6 June 1998, Late Edition, Sec A, p. 6). Even on the initial disclosure of the operation it seemed reasonably clear that the undercover operation violated Mexican law and sovereignty as well as several bilateral co-operation agreements (ibid.).

According to the *New York Times* (11 June 1998, Sec. A, p. 1), this operation began after US Customs officials noticed suspicious transactions involving Mexican bank drafts drawn on US dollar accounts held in the United States. The original observations of these suspicious transactions were made in 1993 and by 1995 a full-scale operation was under way headed by a senior US Customs official named William F. Gately. The details of the Operation Casablanca case are mired in controversy, claims and counter-claims, but some of the facts seem well established enough to use it to highlight the dangers that undercover sting operations entail. What seems clear is that US Customs did uncover a substantial money-laundering operation and the arrest of 142 suspects, the confiscation of US $35 million and the freezing of US $66 million more, reported in the *New York Times* (16 March 1999, Sec. A, p. 1) amply confirm this. Several details of the case, however, are salient and indicative of the problematic nature of such operations. Gately himself apparently came extremely close to being a rogue agent. A former US marine who had volunteered for service in Vietnam at the age of 17, Gately had developed a reputation among Customs agents and the US law enforcement community generally for risky business. He had cast himself in the mould of a lonely crusader with a deep sense of mission, surrounded by small-minded bureaucrats. At one point during the unfolding of the case it emerged that John Hensley, Gately's supervisor at the US Customs office in Los Angeles, had accused him of transgressions ranging from travelling without authorisation to stealing millions of dollars, but these suggestions were later dismissed as baseless by the Customs Commissioner, Raymond W. Kelly, some time after Gately's retirement (*New York Times*, 19 March 1999, Sec. A, p. 1). Gately's operation uncovered an extensive money-laundering operation that putatively extended up to the highest levels of the Mexican government. He maintained that it included the highest levels of the Mexican military and even suggested that

President Zedillo was involved, but he was never able to produce concrete evidence of this. When Operation Casablanca was drawn to a close, Gately claimed that the action was premature and that higher officials could have been drawn into the net and more money confiscated. 'Why are we sitting on this information?', he asked, 'It's either because we're lazy, we're stupid or the political will doesn't exist to engage in the kind of investigation where our law enforcement efforts might damage our foreign policy' (*New York Times*, 16 March 1999, Sec. A, p. 1). On 25 March the *New York Times* (Sec. A, p. 6) quoted both Hensley and Kelly (Gately's superiors) to the effect that statements reported in that paper the previous week, and widely interpreted as suggesting that senior Clinton Administration officials had improperly declined to extend the life of the investigation, amounted to 'a significant allegation'. Mr Kelly stated that the charge that the case was brought to a close 'so that US officials could keep a high-ranking Mexican Government official from being investigated as part of the case is grossly untrue and irresponsible'.

The case attracted notoriety for reasons other than the fractiousness exposed within the ranks of the US law-enforcement apparatus. The operation had been kept secret from Mexican officials at all levels of government. One US official, who declined to be named, had a very negative reaction when Gately outlined the details of his plans for the undercover sting. He recalled stating bluntly: 'You must be out of your mind' (*New York Times*, 16 March 1999, Sec. A, p. 1). It emerged during the course of a trial in the Federal District Court in Los Angeles (which returned a split verdict, convicting three Mexican bankers and acquitting three others), that the case was largely dependent on a 'co-operating informant', Fred Mendoza (alias Javier Ramirez) (*New York Times*, 10 June 1999, Sec. A, p. 30). Mendoza had already been paid US $2.3 million and stood to gain a further US $7.5 million under the terms of a 'personal service agreement' he had agreed with US Customs. It is notable that law enforcement officials also admitted during the trial that even these large sums of money did not make him the highest-paid informer US law enforcement agencies had ever employed (*New York Times*, 29 April 1999, Sec. A, p. 18). The lucrative business of being a criminal informant provoked much comment, but what stood out most about Mendoza was his extensive previous criminal involvement, documented back to as early as 1989. In court he admitted to helping with the arrangements to ship 1,320 pounds of cocaine in 1992. It also emerged in court that Mendoza had turned informant after an incident with another group of cocaine smugglers in which he was abducted and threatened over a debt owed by his brother, a drug

trafficker who also worked for US Customs. Admissions regarding the
depth of dependence that Operation Casablanca owed to Mendoza's
penetration of the clandestine cocaine trade and the money laundering associated with it seemed to contradict earlier claims by Customs
officials that they had not approached any bankers; 'They all came to
us' (*New York Times*, 20 May 1998, Sec. A, p. 6).

It remains difficult to comprehend all the facets of Operation Casablanca and details are likely to continue emerging as the legal process
continues to wind its way through the US court system. Alejandro
Mayorkas, the United States Attorney in Los Angeles, and Duane
Lyons, the chief prosecutor in the case, have declined to comment on
the verdicts thus far handed down, citing the pending forfeiture phase
of the case (*New York Times*, 11 June 1999, Sec. A, p. 30). This phase
may reveal other aspects of the case that are an embarrassment to
American officials. Operation Casablanca undoubtedly soured relations between the USA and Mexico. For example, Mexico continues
be refuse broad diplomatic immunity to US agents operating on their
territory, something that US officials have been attempting to negotiate
for years (*New York Times*, 11 June 1998, Sec. A, p. 1) and Mexican
officials complained loudly of the infringement of their sovereignty.
Citing the close co-operation between Mexican authorities and both
the DEA and FBI, Mexican officials argued that they could have helped
to expose a much wider part of the same drug organisation. The operation certainly exposed tensions within the US government itself after it
was revealed that not only was the Mexican Government not informed
about the operation, but also that senior officials at the White House,
the State Department and even the Treasury Department were kept in
the dark (ibid.). Secretary of State Madeleine Allbright was one of
several officials who were sharply critical, stating in a letter to Treasury
Secretary Robert Rubin, in part, that 'we might have achieved more
favorable results if we had brought Attorney General Madrazo and a
few others into our confidence . . . I do not wish to interfere with your
law enforcement work, but I do believe we need to do a better job of
coordination' (ibid.). The irony is that Operation Casablanca might not
have been necessary at all. In the midst of the diplomatic furore that
emerged in the immediate aftermath of the first public announcements
regarding the operation, and continued during the court proceedings,
the Mexican and US governments were actively trading witnesses in
the pursuit of drug-related corruption. Indeed, at their own initiative,
Mexican officials had arranged to bring Adrian Carrera Fuentes to
Houston on 3 June 1998 to give testimony against Ruiz Massieu, Raul
Salinas and others close to the Mexican President. This testimony had

been scheduled before the diplomatic uproar over Operation Casablanca (*New York Times*, 15 July 1998, Sec. A, p. 1). Mexican co-operation in this regard continued to be forthcoming in spite of the much-soured atmosphere produced by the revelations surrounding the undercover initiative.

Martha Cottam and Otwin Marenin (1999) have noted the American 'colonial image of Mexico', which puts the USA in a 'masters of the universe' position *vis-à-vis* Mexico which must be kept supine. They contrast this with a Mexican nationalism jealous of encroachment on her sovereignty as the crucial explanatory factor in the difficult working relations between the two countries. Peter Andreas (1996, 1997) has argued a stronger case, that the effects of the free-market reforms associated with the North American Free Trade Agreement (NAFTA), together with drug prohibition, has 'narcotized' the Mexican state and turned the USA into a 'Crimefare State', thus creating the twin effects of corruption and cloak-and-dagger and militarised law enforcement that characterise policing in the region. According to Deputy Attorney-General Jamie E. Gorelick, speaking in 1996, the foreign efforts of US law enforcement agents are a simple extension of US domestic law enforcement: 'all we are doing is following cases here in the United States to their origins abroad . . . so we're performing a very traditional law enforcement function; it just takes us into foreign countries' (cited in Andreas 1997: 40). This is extra-territorial law enforcement which, because of its straightforward transgressions of sovereignty, is something rather different to true transnational policing.

What this case amply illustrates is the inherent danger of duplicity in undercover operations. Things do not always go according to plan, and even when they do, the ramifications may be felt far away from where the plans were originally hatched. When 'deep cover' operations are mounted, these dangers are multiplied manyfold. Further, when such operations are transnational and involve several agencies it is not always possible to see who is accountable for decisions taken. Operation Casablanca illustrates this point, but there are other examples. For instance, in the course of the parliamentary inquiry following the so-called IRT scandal in the Netherlands,[12] it was not possible for the select committee to question DEA agents who may have been in a position to provide some insight into the undercover operations that gave rise to the scandal, because they claimed diplomatic immunity (den Boer 1997; Sheptycki 1999). Further, the cross-national and inter-agency nexus in which police agents operate, creates a collage of procedural rules and regulations which are not necessarily commensurate with each other; this is revealed in the Chinoy case. In Chinoy ([1992]

1 All ER 317, D.C.; WCHR No. 15199/89) the US Drug Enforcement Agency undertook a telephone wiretap in France without the authorisation of a local *juge d' instruction* (investigating magistrate, whose job it is to oversee all aspects of police investigations). This was in breach of French law and a violation of her sovereignty as well as being, arguably, in breach of the European Human Rights Convention. A case for extradition was subsequently brought in the UK and evidence taken from this wiretap was admitted in court. The decision to grant the request for extradition was based largely on this evidence and was eventually upheld by the European Court of Human Rights. Were the police agents pursuing this case to have tried to introduce this evidence in a French court it would certainly have been disregarded on procedural grounds (Gane and Mackarel 1996).[13]

Nor is this an isolated instance. 'Jurisdiction shopping' appears to be a common feature of transnational police operations (Sheptycki 1996). Studies have shown that, where possible, arrests will be made in jurisdictions which have procedural rules which are the most amenable to the law enforcement case. This is what Professor Peter Tak meant when he suggested that if the Dutch criminal justice system tried to tighten up the procedural rules for undercover operations 'to escape from strict rules the Dutch police will push suspects abroad' (quoted in Sheptycki 1999: 18; see also Klerks 1995; Tak 1997). Tak had already noted that the legal controls for undercover operations in France and Germany were looser than they were in the Netherlands. Thus amelioration of perceived problems in the Dutch police system could not be solved by simply 'putting their own house in order'. This suggests a trend whereby concerted pressure from the law enforcement community to tackle international organised crime results in procedural law moving in the direction of the lowest common denominator. Neither are these concerns confined to procedural rules, since it has been suggested that in some instances police have sought to bring cases to trial on the basis of calculating which national jurisdiction is likely to hand out the more severe penalty (Sheptycki 1996: 61).

Nadelmann (1993) outlined the evolution of undercover operations in Europe, where in the period following World War II there grew up a marked (and understandable) dislike of undercover police methods. The evolutionary process was such that the DEA and some European police agents responded to legal prohibitions on the use of such techniques, first by employing them anyway, then by persuading and pressuring prosecutors to sanction their use and, ultimately, by inducing judges and legislators to legalise the practices (p. 236). Nadelmann argued that European courts, legislators and the authors of internal police guidelines tended to respond to perceived inadequacies in the legal frame for policing transnational organised crime by expanding police power and discretion. In short, pressures arise from the need to legalise and regulate what the police have already begun to do 'extra-legally' (p. 248). It has been further argued that the evolution towards 'increased international co-operation between authorities tends to disturb the fragile balance between prosecution and defence in a criminal case' (Harding et al. 1995: 103; see also, Sheptycki 1997). Thus, while multilateral and bilateral legal instruments have evolved to facilitate the prosecution in the trial process (by the provision of evidence, transfer of proceedings, extradition and so on) there has been no comparable advance to facilitate the defence. Christopher Harding and Bert Swart thus argued that those who stand accused of transnational crime will need to acquire rights to transnational legal co-operation to the extent necessary for a proper legal defence and they suggest that the right to compel the attendance of witnesses from abroad might be such a right (Harding et al. 1995: 103). So, even where rules which rationalise the legal frame for criminal law enforcement have been put in place, these do not necessarily operate without systemic bias. Harding and Swart pointed out that 'abuse of power or errors committed by national authorities in one state almost never entail legal consequences in another state', that is: 'most courts in Europe are not prepared to attach consequences to illegal behaviour by officials other than those of their own country' (p. 104).

A pattern seems evident in the evolution of transnational criminal law enforcement whereby the legal advantage has been put in the law enforcement camp. This is strikingly at odds with the position put forward by police themselves, which usually suggests that the balance is in favour of the law breakers. It seems clear that the attempt to ensure that national frontiers do not present obstacles to police has led to a consistent loosening of the legal structure that police investigations should, in theory, operate under (Passas and Groskin 1995: 303–4), at least according to the 'due process model' (Packer 1968).[14] Further, it appears that this loosening is occurring at least partly in the wake of extra-legal action by law enforcement. Even in states where international standards laid down in such instruments as the International Covenant on Civil and Political Rights or the European Convention on Human Rights are broadly accepted, the rights of suspects and affected third parties are treated in a variety of ways which are inconsistent and not wholly in accord with the spirit of human rights legislation. During the course of this legal evolution it appears that little thought was given to the issues surrounding the arrest of foreign nationals and their incarceration in a state not their own, or to questions about the adequate provision of legal counsel for such persons and the availability of bail where appropriate. With regard to money laundering specifically, there are few enabling mechanisms for effective challenges to be made to asset freezing or forfeiture orders which have often been made *ex parte*. Moreover, standards of proof are not uniform in all states and there seems to be an international trend towards lowering the standard of proof necessary in such cases.[15]

The development of a transnational anti-money-laundering regime is evidently shaped by a number of factors related to the nature of the institutional actors. The actions of states, bilaterally or multilaterally, have a significant effect, as do certain transnational institutions which 'govern at a distance' (that is above) sovereign states (most notably the G7 and the OECD, and their offspring the FATF). Private institutions such as banks and the like also shape the regime. The vested interest of financial institutions in maintaining aspects of confidentiality is conditioned by the fact that unrestricted access by state officials to banking and other financial records would very plausibly encourage capital flight to more permissive jurisdictions and that capital flight need not be restricted to 'dirty money'. The consequence of these competing interests appears to be the development of a 'hybrid system of governance' (O'Malley 1999), whereby criminal law enforcement and prudential regulation both provide opportunities for control. Law enforcement remains pre-eminent in some respects, not least because of the sanctioning of such techniques as the 'sting operation'. The practices of what are essentially sub-state institutions thus have a considerable effect on the quality and nature of transnational governance.

Clandestine markets and the illicit life of electronic money

Money has become a global artefact and the keystone of an economic structure that straddles the world. As we enter the cyber-age, e-money dominates the economic systems of production, ownership, labour and consumption, heralding the 'age of money' (Weatherford 1997). The emergence of the global electronic money system with currencies floating freely against each other allows millions of dollars to be transferred from one currency to another instantly and incessantly every minute of every day of the year. In 1995 it was estimated that this homeless money had surpassed the US $1.3 trillion a day mark. Criminologists, together with other social theorists, have noted that, given the mobility of electronic money, states can no longer expect to control or direct its flows and this has given rise to a suggestion of the 'hollowing out of the state' (Giddens 1990; Bottoms and Wiles 1995; Sheptycki 1995; Castells 1997). The thesis, stated briefly, is this: the mercurial transience of capital in the circuits of the global financial system has removed the power of decision-making to a macro-level beyond that of the state. According to this logic, market forces, not political majorities, now compel the reconfiguration of societies that nation-states vainly try to circumscribe. As Bottoms and Wiles (1997) put it '[the] ability of nation states to control this transnational capital and business is not very great, precisely because they do not operate solely within the territory of a nation state' (p. 350). In part they conclude that 'the main definers of crime [policy-makers nestled within the nation-state] . . . will cede their power . . . upwards to transnational capital and political organisations' (pp. 349–50). Others have suggested that the days of the nation-state system are numbered as the tax base is gradually eroded by the tides of electronic money and they even welcome this development (Davidson and Rees-Mogg 1997). Studies displaying great erudition are no less pessimistic, as Jack Weatherford observed in *The History of Money* (1997). In the emerging global economy the power of money and the institutions built will come to supersede that of any nation, combination of nations, or international organisations. He felt compelled to conclude that 'propelled and pro-tected by the power of electronic technology, a new global elite is emerging – an elite without loyalty to any particular country' (p. 268).

Contemporary developments in anti-money laundering reveal that state agents are not so impotent in the transnational realm as this picture describes. Legitimate markets are like clandestine ones, players in them seek to maximise the value of their wealth and they do not always want to do so in ways that the authorities can account for. Insofar as players in both of these markets operate within the trans-national financial system, they operate at a remove from state author-ities and many analysts have naturally focused on the de-coupling or dis-embedding of capital (legitimate and illicit) from the nation-state. The hollowing out of the state thesis is a product of this train of thought. However, the idea of 'hitting criminals where it hurts . . . in the bank balance', has supplied police agencies from the G7 and/or OECD nations with investigative techniques backed by a powerful moral logic that allows them the access necessary to patrol the circuits of global finance. The resulting anti-money laundering regime can be characterised as government (or governance) at a distance. Actions of the G7, the OECD, the FATF and a host of other transnational insti-tutions which represent the interests of seigneurial sovereign states in the world system are concrete instances of this. The recent emergence of the Egmont Group in Europe and SWIFT globally are practical steps towards transnational exchange of financial and banking information which show that distanciated governmental practices at the sub-national, national and transnational level can be brought into an elaborate *opus araneum*.[16] It has been argued that the development of this transnational regime of governance is necessary because the global financial system is so susceptible to crises arising from systemic volatility. The enormity of illicit funds circulating in the transnational banking and financial system represents an unacceptable level of risk to a febrile world economy which is almost too hot to handle (Pieth 1998: 161). Prophylactic efforts to prevent the passage of 'dirty money' into the global banking network are thus not only calculated to salvage the reputations of banking systems vulnerable to the charge that they are colluding with criminal entrepreneurs, such measures serve to protect them against the miasma of illicit capital itself. Criminal money threatens the global financial system by eroding norms and standards of conduct – prudential control of the kind advocated by the FATF is therefore good preventative medicine. Undertaking such control measures through criminal law enforcement 'sting operations', the techniques of forensic accountancy and self-policing measures such as the prudential surveillance increasingly practised in the offshore banking world (under the oversight of the FATF) do not so much indicate a 'hollowing out of the state', but rather a diffusion, multiplication and intensification of governmental practice, from within certain specific sovereign states outwards, from the transnational level downwards and from sub-state institutions upwards. However, this 'polycentricity' of power (Stenson 1999) creates uncertainties about the accountability of global governance.

It could be plausibly argued that action against drug money is a governmental 'Trojan Horse', and that the surveillance systems currently being installed in the transnational finance system, which aim to seek out the money launderers working on behalf of criminal enterprise can be converted to target the potentially bigger prizes squirreled away by tax evaders. For example, currently tax evasion remains a civil offence in Switzerland, although the federal prosecutor Carla del Ponte, who has worked to lessen Swiss bank secrecy laws, has also indicated a desire to make it a criminal offence (*The Economist*, 28 March 1998). The UNDCP noted in its report in 1998 that 'it cannot be said that Switzerland rolls out the welcome mat for drug money' but money 'deriving from tax and exchange control evasion is quite another matter' (1998: 9). The fine line between tax avoidance and tax evasion may be shifting. Indeed, in announcing the review of financial regulation in the Channel Islands and the Isle of Man that produced the Edwards Report, the UK Home Secretary Jack Straw stated that, with regard to criminal investigations, the review would examine 'collaboration between the island authorities and overseas authorities in investigating suspected financial crime, including fiscal offences', that is: tax evasion (Stuart 1998). Governments lose considerable revenue from corporate taxes due to the advent of the global economy and have done so since the first multinationals took advantage of their transnational business relations to escape national tax systems (Tugendhat 1971). A more recent recognition is that the globalisation of finance has eroded government's ability to tax individuals, especially 'high net-worth individuals'. It has become harder to tax personal income because professional workers are more mobile than they were two decades ago. Even if individuals do not become tax exiles, many earn a growing slice of their income overseas and such income is relatively easy to hide in an offshore haven. Taxing personal savings and the income from speculative investment also becomes harder when the circuits of global finance allow private wealth to be moved across the globe (*The Economist*, 31 May 1997). Globalisation of banking and finance has demonstrably undermined governmental ability to raise tax revenues from individuals and corporations, either by making evasion easier, or by encouraging economic activity to shift to lower-tax countries. Thus it has been observed that 'Governments around the world, from India to the United States, from Argentina to Russia, are finding that they are losing much of the tax revenue due under their laws because of the calculated use of foreign secrecy. The situation is so bad that the opportunity to commit the crime of tax evasion is advertised openly on the internet by hundreds of firms' (UNDCP 1998: 70–1). The surveillance system installed in the circuits of the global financial system – making bankers, accountants and lawyers responsible for reporting suspicious transactions (or risk criminal prosecution) may well be a technique of governance at a distance which could eventually enable world-wide tax collection on behalf of national sovereign states.

Validation of the 'Trojan Horse hypothesis' awaits future developments. Its plausibility suggests that the 'hollowing out of the state' may well be chimerical, a temporary state of affairs, or due to other factors altogether (such as the embrace of neo-liberal ideology). But one important counter-argument needs to be mentioned and addressed. Much of the literature describing the problems relating to 'dirty money' and the transnational efforts to control money laundering emphasise the enormity of the task and the relatively puny institutional strength of the governmental controllers. 'The offshore financial world is appropriately described as a "Bermuda Triangle" for investigations of money-laundering, complex financial fraud and tax evasion', warn the scientific advisors to the United Nations Office for Drug Control and Crime Prevention. 'Money trails disappear, connections are obscured and investigations encounter so many obstacles that they are often abandoned' (UNDCP 1998: 33).

This suggests that the existing transnational anti-money-laundering regime is taking on a task no less daunting than the one foisted upon Sisyphus. The inference might be that the apparent weakness of the controllers *vis-à-vis* the hot money managers is conclusive evidence of a weakening of state power in the transnational era and, by implication, as evidence of 'hollowing out of the state'. This counterargument might melt away, at least in the view of some, if we note that the governmental project has been 'congenitally failing' since the dawn of modernity (cf. Miller and Rose 1990). Certainly the 'congenital failure' of governmental efforts are observable across a whole range of strategies aimed at fostering drug law prohibition at the neighbourhood, municipal, provincial, national, regional or global level (see chapter seven). Looked at this way, failure to create total control in the global financial system is but one more instance in the practice of governance. Congenital failure is quite likely to manifest itself with regard to the global anti-money-laundering regime, especially as the effects of new information technologies continue to make themselves felt. Notable here are two developments: encryption and stored value systems. Encryption will allow the use of the internet in global money management and the traditional underground banking systems of the Middle and Far East (noted earlier in this chapter) are just two of the mechanisms that will gain strength from these developments. Stored value systems offer yet another way for financial transactions to escape the surveillance systems of transnational governance (Grabosky and Smith 1998). Perhaps the fluidity of electronic money really will undermine the structure of the state system after all.

Regardless of the explanatory power that either the 'hollowing out of the state hypothesis' or the 'Trojan Horse hypothesis' may be deemed to hold, one point seems indisputable: a law enforcement capacity is evolving in the interstices of the emerging transnational state system that has, as its declared *raison d'être,* the control of clandestine or illicit capital: 'dirty money'. Since this transnational state-system is functioning with a fragmented legal apparatus, law enforcement is not so much performed under the rule of law, but rather employs legal rules instrumentally on the basis of opportunity. At the same time, nation-states are not yielding up social and political power to the emergent transnational realm, but are working to retain sovereign power through intergovernmental means. Transnational policing is thus shaped by three factors: a fragmented legal frame and the consequent weak purview of legal norms; a priority of desperation (especially coming from geopolitically dominant states) that asserts that state sovereign power must be preserved; and a moral logic which provides the justification for the extra-territorial extension of formerly nationally bounded police institutions into the transnational realm. This is a potent mix and there is seemingly no democratic mechanism to guide the process.

What are the likely developments for transnational policing in the financial sphere as we enter the twenty-first century? It is of course impossible to divine what the future may hold with any certainty. It is possible to say that policing emerged as the processes of modern governance developed and, insofar as policing institutions have been embedded in a democratic political context, the practices of policing have struck a fine balance between the interests of individual citizens and those of larger social systems. In the contemporary period social systems transgress national boundaries and so policing systems are extending their reach, consequently operating in a fragmented legal frame. Moreover, mechanisms for ensuring the democratic accountability of transnational policing practices are not being laid in the emerging transnational state system. This raises important questions of principle which are likely to come to the fore as incidents of law enforcement malpractice come to light. What has been shown here is that one of the principal extensions of policing power into the transnational realm in the contemporary period has been in the area of money laundering; the techniques of asset seizure available to police, transnational and otherwise, are therefore likely to produce these test cases. With regard to the development of the anti-money-laundering regime, the transnational police enterprise is frequently justified on the basis of the needs of the 'international community' (UNDCP 1998). A rounded assessment of the Global *Gesellschaft* is beyond the boundaries of the analysis pursued here, but we might end by citing the historian of money, Jack Weatherford, who notes that the age of electronic money 'promises to increase even more the role of money in our public and private lives, surpassing kinship, religion, occupation and citizenship as the defining element of social life' (1997: 268). In conditions of such overwhelming anomie the notion of a 'global community' seems quite dubious. Further, policing without the support of the policed has long been recognised as a fruitless exercise, making it doubtful that even the most rigorous law enforcement can clean up the virtual launderette.

Dour prognostications aside, we shall simply have wait to see what comes out in the wash.

Notes

1 The author would like to express thanks to W. C. Gilmore, Dawn Bennett, and Valsamis Mitsilegas for sharing their knowledge about money laundering and the development of international criminal law that pertains to it. A version of this paper was presented at the 17th International Symposium on Economic Crime, Jesus College, Cambridge, 14 September 1999.

2 See Sheptycki 1998a, which contains a case analysis pertaining to the seizure of instruments of high monetary value in the English Channel region.

3 The Society of World-wide Interbank Financial Telecommunications (SWIFT) broadcast a message to its users in the mid-1990s requesting similar recording to take place. Note that this is a request rather than a requirement (Drage 1993). SWIFT is the primary mechanism for international financial transactions, but to date there is no data on its operational success in anti-money-laundering efforts.

4 Reportedly, neither the futures and securities markets nor insurance and pensions were much used to launder money when these early efforts to control money laundering were mounted (Gilmore 1995: 45; Parlour 1995: 283–4). As surveillance of the bank system tightened, money-laundering activity was displaced to other parts of the financial system, see below.

5 Two more US federal statutes were created in 1970 to deal with drug trafficking and organized crime: the Racketeer Influenced and Corrupt Organizations Act (RICO) and the Continuing Criminal Enterprise (CCE) statute.

6 Not all of these cases involve criminal acts. Consider the case of one well respected Alabama physician. In 1992, acting on the suggestion of close friends who had opened a new local bank, the doctor requested his current banker to transfer his life savings (about US $2.6 million) to the new institution. He did not know or understand about the need to file a Currency Transaction Report (CTR), nor did his attorney or any of the bankers involved inform him of his duty to file. Failing to file a CTR is a felony offence punishable by a $250,000 fine and up to five years in jail. Additionally, his entire life savings were at risk of being forfeited to the US government. Understandably, he decided to fight the charges on the grounds that his money was legitimately obtained and that the failure to file was merely an administrative oversight. In taking this action his lawyer argued that, were the savings in question much smaller, the authorities would not have had the financial incentive to seize them. The Internal Revenue Service (IRS) subsequently placed liens on all of his assets and property and, with no ready cash available, he was unable to pay his income taxes when they came due. The Department of Justice filed an additional charge against him of 'conspiracy to obstruct justice'. At his 1995 trial in US District Court, the doctor was acquitted of all the charges against him. The court returned his $2.6 million savings and he settled his problems with the IRS, but the affair cost him several hundred thousand dollars in legal fees.

170   *James Sheptycki*

7 In one of the cases before the Supreme Court, a Michigan man forfeited the value of his house because he was found to have possessed marijuana there. In this case, there was never any intimation that the individual had used the proceeds of crime to buy his house, nor was it shown that the drugs in his possession were ever intended for use by anyone other than himself. This case was not an isolated instance.

8 The $750 figure was reportedly established on the basis of studies that showed that immigrants working in the United States sent money home to their families in amounts of less than $500 (LEN, No. 468, 1997).

9 In one instance the Bank of Nova Scotia in Grand Cayman refused to disclose details of an account as requested by the United States Internal Revenue Service. When the President of that bank landed in New York to change planes *en route* to Canada he was arrested and detained until the bank provided the information requested.

10 Membership of the FATF was closed in the mid-1990s as expansion beyond 26 members was deemed to have the potential to compromise its efficiency and effectiveness. Those member states are: Australia, Austria, Belgium, Canada, Denmark, Finland, France, Germany, Greece, Hong Kong, Iceland, Ireland, Italy, Japan, Luxembourg, The Netherlands, New Zealand, Norway, Portugal, Singapore, Spain, Sweden, Switzerland, Turkey, the United Kingdom and the United States. Additionally the Commission of the European Communities and the Gulf Co-operation Council also had representation. In the late 1990s the FATF had developed two 'regional groups', the Caribbean FATF and the Asia–Pacific Group, signalling the establishment of 'an international network of regional organisations' rather than 'one large global organisation' (Smith, 1998, p. 8).

11 The actual extent of this displacement has not been empirically verified. The withdrawal, in the face of industry pressure, of 'Know Your Customer' legislation in the United States in March 1999, which had been put forward by the US Federal Reserve, suggests that displacement pressure might have been a chimera of governmental programmers rather than a significant problem for the financial industry. This legislation would have greatly enhanced the legal requirements for due diligence and suspicious activity reporting, practices which were already entrenched as best practice in the United States anyway. Saverio Mirarchi, vice-president in charge of anti-money laundering compliance at the American Express Company head office in New York, noted a tension between the needs of government and the ideals of client confidentiality in his presentation to the 17th International Symposium on Economic Crime at Jesus College, Cambridge, in September 1999. According to him, while money service businesses like AmEx were keen to ensure the propriety of transactions undertaken through their systems, there had been 'very little analysis of the cost imposed on institutions in doing this surveillance' and 'very little analysis showing either the benefits to reduce or prevent crime or to protect the [money services] institutions'. There also remained questions about who should pay: the tax-payer, the financial institutions or their customers. In the final analysis, according to Mirarchi, 'confidentiality rules are part of broader legal principles about protecting the privacy of individuals [and] as such they are legitimate and desirable'. He also added that confidentiality rules 'should never be used to protect perpetrators of fraud or other criminal activity'.

12 The IRT (inter-regional team) scandal refers to a long-term undercover operation conducted in the Netherlands which ended in ignominy in the early 1990s amidst suggestions that police over-stepped the legal boundaries laid down for the conduct of such operations. See Sheptycki 1999: 17–20 for further details of the parliamentary inquiry that followed.

13 Chinoy is an example of a case where evidence unlawfully obtained abroad is presented to a system which is prepared to accept such evidence in judicial proceedings. Gane and Mackarel (1996) note that, for completeness sake, legal analysis should also take cognisance of the converse instance wherein evidence lawfully obtained abroad is technically inadmissible in the jurisdiction of the court considering the case. They cite a number of cases where evidence obtained from telephone taps undertaken in the Netherlands, France and Sweden was submitted in Belgian courts. In Belgium, evidence from telephone taps was considered, at the time of these cases, to be contrary to domestic law. In the three instances sited by Gane and Mackarel the evidence was accepted after it had been shown to the Belgian court's satisfaction that the evidence-gathering procedures were both in accord with domestic law in the jurisdiction in which the taps were carried out and that the procedures were not in conflict with the European Convention on Human Rights (pp. 113–15).

14 A number of socio-legalists question whether legal regulation has ever directed or circumscribed operational policing. Doreen McBarnet (1981) has argued that the relation is actually the reverse, that law *facilitates* police practice. Richard Ericson (1994) put the matter succinctly when he wrote that 'due process is for crime control' (p. 113). By extension, with respect to transnational police operations, in an operational context which takes place within multiple jurisdictions (a fragmented legal frame), police may pick and choose which 'due process' rules to invoke, which further extends the scope for pursuit of 'crime control' aims.

15 In late 1998 the UK Home Secretary proposed a major extension of civil forfeiture. He proposed a new agency, The National Confiscation Agency, whose job it would be to ask civil courts to decide on 'the balance of probabilities' if a given suspect's wealth had been legitimately earned. Up to this point asset forfeiture was decided on the more stringent requirements of the criminal law: 'beyond reasonable doubt'. However, the proposed changes to the UK system still fell short of the US and Hong Kong systems where the burden of proof falls on suspects to show that their wealth has been legitimately acquired rather than on the state to prove wrongdoing (Steele 1988; Rufford 1998).

16 Literally 'spider's work' a term that describes a type of intricate lace-work which resembles a spider's web. Thanks to Sarah Sheptycki for suggesting this variation on Stan Cohen's now classic criminological metaphor of 'netwidening' (Cohen 1985).

References

Andreas, P. (1996) 'Narcotizing the State and Economy in Mexico: Side-Effects of Free Market Reform and Drug Market Prohibition', unpublished paper presented at the International Law and Society Meetings, Glasgow, 10–13 July 1996.

Andreas, P. (1997) 'The Rise of the American Crimefare State', *World Policy Journal*, Fall, pp. 37–44.

Arlacchi, P. (1993) 'Corruption, Organized Crime and Money Laundering World Wide', in M. Punch (ed.), *Coping with Corruption in a Borderless World*, Deventer: Kluwer.

Arrasia, J. (1996) 'Money Laundering – A US Perspective', in B. Rider and M. Ashe (eds), *Money Laundering Control*, Dublin: Round Hall, Sweet and Maxwell.

Bamber, D. (1998) 'Straw to Tighten Money Rules on Channel Isles', *Sunday Telegraph*, 1 November.

den Boer, M. (1997) *Undercover Policing and Accountability from an International Perspective*, Maastricht: European Institute of Public Administration.

Bottoms, A. and Wiles, P. (1995) 'Crime and Insecurity in the City', in C. Fijnaut, J. Goethals, T. Peters and L. Walgrave (eds), *Changes in Society: Crime and Criminal Justice in Europe* (2 vols), The Hague: Kluwer.

Bottoms, A. and Wiles, P. (1997) 'Environmental Criminology', in M. Maguire, R. Morgan and R. Reiner (eds), *The Oxford Handbook of Criminology*, Oxford: Clarendon Press.

Bridges, M. (1996) 'Tax Evasion – A Crime in Itself: The Relationship with Money Laundering', *Journal of Financial Crime*, Vol. 4, No. 2.

Castells, M. (1997) *The Power of Identity*, Oxford: Basil Blackwell.

Cohen, S. (1985) *Visions of Social Control*, Cambridge: Polity Press.

Commonwealth Law Bulletin (1992) 'Editorial Note on United States vs Alvarez-Machain: State Sponsored Kidnapping in Lieu of Extradition', Vol. 18, pp. i–iii.

Cottam, M. and Marenin, O. (1999) 'International Co-operation in the War on Drugs: Mexico and the United States', *Policing and Society*, Vol. 9, No. 3, pp. 209–40.

Cressey, D. R. (1969) *Theft of a Nation: The Structure and Operations of Organized Crime in America*, New York: Harper and Row.

Cullen, P. (1993) 'Money Laundering: The European Community Directive', pp. 34–49 in H. MacQueen (ed.) *Money Laundering, Hume Papers on Public Policy*, Vol. 1, No. 2.

Davidson, J. D. and Rees Mogg, W. (1997) *The Sovereign Individual*, London: Macmillan.

Drage, J. (1993) 'Countering Money Laundering: the Response of the Financial Sector', in H. MacQueen (ed.), *Money Laundering, Hume Papers on Public Policy*, Vol. 1, No. 2, Edinburgh: Edinburgh University Press.

Ericson, R. V. (1994) 'The Royal Commission on Criminal Justice System Surveillance', in M. McConville and L. Bridges (eds), *Criminal Justice in Crisis*, Aldershot: Edward Elgar.

Fijnaut, C. and Marx, G. (1995) *Undercover: Police Surveillance in Comparative Perspective*, The Hague: Kluwer.

Gane, C. and Mackarel, M. (1996) 'The Admissibility of Evidence Obtained from Abroad into Criminal Proceedings – the Interpretation of Mutual

Legal Assistance Treaties and Use of Evidence Irregularly Obtained', *European Journal of Crime, Criminal Law and Criminal Justice*, Vol. 4, No. 2, pp. 98–119.

Garland, D. (1996) 'The Limits of the Sovereign State: Strategies of Crime Control in Contemporary Society', *British Journal of Criminology*, Vol. 36, No. 4, pp. 445–71.

Garland, D. (1997) 'The Punitive Society: Penology, Criminology and the History of the Present', *Edinburgh Law Review*, Vol. 1, No. 2, pp. 180–200.

Garland, D. (1999) 'Governmentality and the Problem of Crime', in R. Smandych (ed.), *Governable Places: Reading on Governmentality and Crime Control*, Aldershot: Ashgate.

Giddens, A. (1990) *The Consequences of Modernity*, Cambridge: Polity Press.

Gilmore, W. C. (1991) *Combating International Drugs Trafficking: The 1988 United Nations Convention against Illicit Traffic in Narcotic Drugs and Psychotropic Substances, Explanatory Documentation*, London: Commonwealth Secretariat.

Gilmore, W. C. (1993) 'Money Laundering: the International Aspect', pp. 1–11 in H. MacQueen (ed.) *Money Laundering, Hume Papers on Public Policy*, Vol. 1, No. 2.

Gilmore, W. C. (1995) *Dirty Money: The Evolution of Money Laundering Counter-Measures*, 2nd edition 1999, Strasbourg: Council of Europe Press.

Grabosky, P. N. and Smith, R. G. (1998) *Crime in the Digital Age: Controlling Telecommunications and Cyberspace Illegalities*, New Brunswick, NJ: Transaction.

Greenberg, T. (1994) 'Anti-Money Laundering Activities in the United States', *Action Against Transnational Criminality*, Vol. III, *The Proceedings of the 1993 Conference on International White Collar Crime*, London: Commonwealth Secretariat.

Harding, C., Fennell, P., Jörg, N. and Swart, B. (1995) *Criminal Justice in Europe: A Comparative Study*, Oxford: Clarendon Press.

IELR (1995a) 'President Clinton Uses UN for Announcing Initiatives against International Crime', *International Enforcement Law Reporter*, Vol. 13, Issue 12, December, pp. 493–4.

IELR (1995b) '7 Governments Cooperate and Establish Anguillan Bank to Catch Organized Crime Operatives in Colombia and Italy', in *International Enforcement Law Reporter*, Vol. 11, Issue 2, February 1995, pp. 39–42.

IELR (1996) 'Swiss Cabinet Approves Anti-money Laundering Law', *International Enforcement Law Reporter*, Vol. 12, Issue 7, July, p. 254.

IELR (1997a) 'US Proposes Tough Rules for Money Transmitters', *International Enforcement Law Reporter*, Vol. 13, Issue 6, June, p. 222.

IELR (1997b) 'Swiss Lower House Rejects Abolishing Bank Secrecy', *International Enforcement Law Reporter*, Vol. 13, Issue 1, January, p. 6.

IELR (1998) 'Money Laundering and Bank Secrecy: Financial Action Task Force Releases Annual Report', *International Enforcement Law Reporter*, Vol. 14, Issue 8, August, pp. 309–14.

Klerks, P. (1995) 'Covert Policing in the Netherlands', in C. Fijnaut and G. Marx (eds), *Undercover: Police Surveillance in Comparative Perspective*, The Hague: Kluwer.

LEN (1993) 'Asset Seizures Are Punitive, and Thus Must Fit the Crime', *Law Enforcement News*, Vol. 19, No. 383, 30 June.

LEN (1996a) ' "Drug Rings" Knotty Problem: Moving Cash', *Law Enforcement News*, Vol. 22, No. 446, 31 May.

LEN (1996b) 'Supreme Court OK's Asset Forfeiture: Forfeiture Isn't Punishment', *Law Enforcement News*, Vol. 22, No. 448, 30 June.

LEN (1997a) 'Treasury Puts Screws to Drug $$ Transfers', *Law Enforcement News*, Vol. 23, No. 464, 31 March.

LEN (1997b) 'Drug Enforcement to Bank on: Billions in Narco-profits Eyed', *Law Enforcement News*, Vol. 23, No. 467, 15 May.

LEN (1997c) 'Treasury Widens Efforts against Drug Cartels' Billions', *Law Enforcement News*, Vol. 23, No. 468, 31 May.

McBarnet, D. J. (1981) *Conviction: Law, the State and the Construction of Justice*, London: Macmillan.

McClean, D. (1988) 'Mutual Assistance in Criminal Matters: The Commonwealth Initiative', *International and Comparative Law Quarterly*, Vol. 37, pp. 177–90.

McIntosh, M. (1975) *The Organisation of Crime*, London: Macmillan.

Marx, G. (1988) *Undercover: Police Surveillance in America*, Berkeley: University of California Press.

Miller, P. and Rose, N. (1990) 'Governing Economic Life', *Economy and Society*, Vol. 19, No. 1, pp. 1–27.

Ministry of Justice (1992) *Organised Crime in the Netherlands: An Outline of the Threat and the Plan to Tackle It*, The Hague: Ministry of Justice, Ministry of Home Affairs, September 1992.

Morvillo, R. G. and Bohrer, B. A. (1995) 'Checking the Balance: Prosecutorial Power in an Age of Expansive Legislation', *American Criminal Law Review*, Vol. 32, No. 2, pp. 137–56.

Nadelmann, E. (1993) *Cops Across Borders: The Internationalization of US Criminal Law Enforcement*, University Park PA: Pennsylvania University Press.

Nelken, D. (1997) 'The Globalization of Crime and Criminal Justice', in M. D. A. Freeman and A. D. E. Lewis (eds), *Law and Opinion at the End of the Twentieth Century, Current Legal Problems*, Vol. 50, Oxford: Oxford University Press.

OCDE Task Force (1984) *Annual Report of the Organized Crime Drug Enforcement Task Force Program*, Washington DC: Office of the Attorney-General.

O'Malley, P. (1999) 'Governmentality and the Risk Society', *Economy and Society*, Vol. 28, No. 1, pp. 138–48.

Packer, H. (1968) *The Limits of the Criminal Sanction*, Stanford CT: Stanford University Press.

Parlour, R. (ed.) (1995) *Butterworth's International Guide to Money Laundering: Law and Practice*, London: Butterworth.

Passas, N. and Nelken, D. (1993) 'The Thin Line between Legitimate and Criminal Enterprises: Subsidy Frauds in the European Community', *Crime Law and Social Change*, Vol. 19, No. 3, pp. 223–44.

Passas, N. and Groskin, R. B. (1995) 'International Undercover Investigations', in C. Fijnaut and G. Marx (eds), *Undercover: Police Surveillance in Comparative Perspective*, The Hague: Kluwer.

Pieth, M. (1998) 'The Prevention of Money Laundering: A Comparative Analysis', *European Journal of Crime, Criminal Law and Criminal Justice*, Vol. 6, No. 2, pp. 159–60.

Payne, T. E. (1999) 'Civil Forfeiture in Law Enforcement: Cash Register Justice', in J. D. Sewell (ed.), *Controversial Issues in Policing*, Boston: Allyn and Bacon.

Quirk, P. J. (1996) *Macroeconomic Implications of Money Laundering*, Washington DC: International Monetary Fund, June.

Raine, L. P. and Cilluffo, F. J. (eds) (1994) *Global Organized Crime: The New Empire of Evil*, Washington DC: Center for Strategic and International Studies.

Reid, P. M. (1996) 'Money Laundering – An Irish Perspective', in B. Rider and M. Ashe (eds), *Money Laundering Control*, Dublin: Round Hall, Sweet and Maxwell.

Rufford, N. (1998) 'Straw Sets up Agency to Seize "Dirty" Money', *Sunday Times*, 8 November.

Ruggiero, V. (1996) *Organized Crime and Corporate Crime in Europe*, Aldershot: Avebury.

Sheptycki, J. W. E. (1995) 'Transnational Policing and the Makings of a Postmodern State', *British Journal of Criminology*, Vol. 35, No. 4, pp. 613–35.

Sheptycki, J. W. E. (1996) 'Law Enforcement, Justice and Democracy in the Transnational Arena: Reflections on the War on Drugs', *International Journal of the Sociology of Law*, Vol. 24, pp. 61–75.

Sheptycki, J. W. E. (1997) 'Transnationalism, Crime Control and the European State System: A Review of the Literature', *International Criminal Justice Review*, Vol. 7, pp. 130–40.

Sheptycki, J. W. E. (1998a) 'European Policing Routes: An Essay on Transnationalisation, Policing and the Information Revolution', in H. Bruisma and J. G. A. van der Vijver (eds), *Public Safety in Europe*, Twente: International Police Institute.

Sheptycki, J. W. E. (1998b) 'Policing, Postmodernism and Transnationalisation', *British Journal of Criminology*, Vol. 38, No. 3, pp. 485–503.

Sheptycki, J. W. E. (1999) 'Political Culture and Structures of Social Control: Police Related Scandal in the Low Countries in Comparative Perspective', *Policing and Society*, Vol. 9, No. 1, pp. 1–31.

Sherman, T. (1993) 'International Efforts to Combat Money Laundering: The Role of the Financial Action Task Force', *Hume Papers on Public Policy*, Vol. 1, No. 2, pp. 12–33.

Smith, H. (1998) 'Task Force Fights Global Crime Problem', *The Financial Times Fraud Report*, June.

Steele, J. (1998) 'Crime's Mr Bigs to have homes and cash seized', *Daily Telegraph*, 11 November.

Stenson, K. (1999) 'Crime Control, Governmentality and Sovereignty', in R. Smandych (ed.), *Governable Places, Readings on Governmentality and Crime Control*, Aldershot: Dartmouth.

Stuart, S. (1998) 'Getting Tough on Tax Evasion in Offshore UK', *The Financial Times Fraud Report*, March, pp. 14–15.

Tak, P. (1997) 'Should the Dutch Criminal Procedure Adopt Elements of Foreign Systems?', in M. den Boer (ed.), *Undercover Policing and Accountability from an International Perspective*, Maastricht: European Institute of Public Administration, pp. 37–47.

Thony, J.-F. (1996) 'Processing Financial Information in Money Laundering Matters: Financial Intelligence Units', *European Journal of Crime, Criminal Law and Criminal Justice*, Vol. 4, No. 3, pp. 257–82.

Tugendhat, C. (1971) *The Multinationals*, London: Eyre and Spottiswoode.

Tyler, G. (1963) *Combating Organized Crime*, special edition of *The Annals of the American Academy of Political and Social Science*, Vol. 347, May.

United Nations Office for Drug Control and Crime Prevention (UNDCP) (1998) 'Financial Havens, Banking Secrecy and Money-Laundering', in *Crime Prevention and Criminal Justice Newsletter*, UNDCP Technical Series, Issue 8 (Double Issue) Nos. 34 and 35, New York: United Nations.

Weatherford, J. (1997) *The History of Money*, New York: Three Rivers Press.

6 Policing new social spaces[1]

Peter K. Manning

Introduction

Policing is a form of social control, or response to a grievance (Black 1996: 5). It is third-party intervention in the name of authority into social relations, and has a long history pertaining to the control of territories and of people. Indeed, in many ways policing has its origins in the military notion of winning, maintaining and expanding control over ground or territory. In the contemporary 'information age' this aspect must be reconsidered. Considerable literature on policing and on the nature of the state exists, and some important and stylish work articulates origins of relationships between policing and the state (Bayley 1975), and there is a growing amount of published work on transnational policing (Benyon et al. 1993; Fijnaut 1993; Nadelmann 1993; Harding et al. 1995; Sheptycki 1995, 1996, 1997, 1998a and b). However, a considerable portion of this literature is descriptive, is limited to concerns about drug law enforcement, or simply explicates the formal structure of such police organisations and their potential powers (Anderson 1989; Anderson et al. 1995; Harding et al. 1995). These works question connections between authority, territory and policing, conventional wisdom since Weber's tracing of relationships between the state, law and the legitimate use of force (Brewer et al. 1988). What they tend to show is that Weber's analysis will no longer suffice as a guide to systematic empirical work on emerging patterns and processes of transnational policing. Let us consider some of the ambiguities of Weber's formulation.

1 Previous definitions of policing should be reconsidered. Sheptycki (1995) argues correctly that previous definitions of policing imply the existence of a bounded, designated and named territory within which a policing mandate is executed. Recent changes in social

organisation signal that, while quite distinctive national, international and transnational police mandates exist (the map), legally constituted policing organisations and the actual ground to be controlled (the territory), are simultaneously shifting. Nation-states and associated police forces may not map, much less control, the territory they claim governance over.

2   'Territory' and 'control' are not always correlated and this is well dramatised in the case of transnational policing. Control remains a heady mixture of economic power and legal justification, as recent American invasions of Panama, Grenada, and sporadic undeclared war on Iraq, Colombia and in Kosovo well illustrate. In this context it would do to note that, while UN forces were bombing Kosovo in early 1999, delegations were sent from the US to instruct Kosovars in 'democratic policing' (Gall 1999).

3   The role of force in bringing about compliance is subtle, especially when the area or behaviour policed is not within the bounds of a nation-state. Bittner's (1970) notion that policing is the means of distributing situationally applied force defines as essential to policing what is an empirical question. This is even more true at the transnational level. Generally speaking, force is less significant than the threat of such, and symbolic force, threats and words, are as central to much policing as physical or weapons-based coercion. More agencies than the police apply force and, in transnational policing, this may mean quite routine involvement of military and security services which bring with them rather different traditions and customs with regards to coercive action. While policing in the Anglo-American world has traditionally succeeded on the basis of minimal force, there is no guarantee that this model will achieve priority as policing is elevated to the transnational domain. The role of the American armed forces in domestic policing, their international role in drug control, and as 'peacekeepers' obscures the line between domestic, national and international policing mandates. The analytic task thus becomes to explain the conditions under which, and frequency with which, force is applied.

4   The state as a holder of a monopoly on the legitimate use of force is problematic, as even Weber recognised (Rheinstein 1954/1969: 5–10). In the contemporary period, private policing forces outnumber those of the public police, and the armed (and continually arming) American population probably possesses *far* more conventional firepower than do police forces. This balance of terror may be swinging back in favour of the police as they militarise

(Kraska and Kappeler 1997; Haggerty and Ericson 1999). The relations between community 'vigilantes' and state police have particular salience in a number of locations, including Northern Ireland, South Africa and the USA and there is reason to think that the list of policy options being explored by state programmers are being pursued in a variety of transnational forums (Brogden and Shearing 1993; Cohen 1995, 1996). On the other hand, the state's monopoly of policing-type powers has also been ceded in large measure to the 'in-house' security providers of multinational corporations and to private security providers (see Johnston, this volume). Insofar as the sociology of policing does not identify which agencies in a given domain use force and when, it remains impoverished.

5 Global policing, as Sheptycki (1998b) notes, reveals various extensions of the quasi-legitimate application of force across borders in non-war conditions. Furthermore, as Bourdieu (1977) dramatises, the nature of violence is changing. Violence now includes 'symbolic violence', the destruction of meanings, connections, continuity through invisible domination. It should be noted that Bourdieu focuses on the ways domestic institutions blind citizens to the destruction of their own epistemological shelters, or conspire in their own dependency, by legitimising and officially cloaking violence in euphemisms (Bourdieu 1977: 190ff). The application of violence to those who do not share a habitus is less problematic and this has profound implications for the continuing evolution of transnational policing.

6 The concept of property and its protection, a traditional rationale for policing, is changing. It is widely acknowledged that information is property, a commodity to be bought and sold at a cost, a source of conflict, secrecy and competition between corporations, states and individuals. The amplification and magnification of the importance of 'intellectual property' for contemporary capitalism remains unremarked in the literature on policing, and yet it clearly has considerable implications for the police mission. For example, the term 'counterfeiting' is usually taken to relate to the production of illegitimate banknotes, but in the contemporary period police are likely to be exercised by the illegitimate production and distribution of designer clothing, computer software, CDs and other items that have value as 'intellectual property' (cf. Aoki 1998).

These points suggest that much analytic work remains. The *territory* of policing – public and private, national and transnational – has been identified, and I would argue further that the social significance of such changes cannot be truly appreciated without considering fundamental changes in social embeddedness (Giddens 1991). Modern technology permits social relations across vast spaces. Instantaneously mediated communication through sound, pictures, texts, and film links the world in a continuous web of stimuli, information and imagery. The non-verbal nature and immediacy of face-to-face communication is being simulated by computers, and conveyed by video cameras attached to computers (Lee 1999; Wright 1999). Most importantly, on-line trading in commodities and stocks (linked and semi-automated in computer networks) orchestrates in fragile and tumultuous fashion the many stock-markets and credit instruments of the world. Moreover, markets on the internet are burgeoning as are advertising, pay-to-access sites, and on-line services. This is possible because all forms of information (sound, pictures, texts, graphics and numbers, for example) can be digitised and transmitted variously. This means that previous labels for machines – recorders, televisions, computers, radios, VCRs, and telephone – are reifications since modes of transmitting and receiving are in flux, being collapsed, combined and reduced in size. These forces render the symbolic, the material and the ideal interchangeably real rather than distinctive.

Clearly, as transformations in information processing proceed, as they are accelerated, minimised and made cheaper, patterns of social control will be modified and reshaped. Newly emergent social spaces will be made meaningful, for a time, by recourse to pre-existing notions, labels and practices, which will be modified as the circulation of symbols and information increasingly becomes electronic and digital. Thus regulation, the ordering of social life by political means, encounters information. These several developments in the nature of communication and social relations, law and territorial sovereignty, are all reflected in policing. What is needed is a conception of policing in the information age, an age in which national boundaries are less marked and clear, where information is a commodity, and secrecy and security concerns are located, in large part, in transnational information networks.

We should also take cognisance of the fact that the rise of transnational policing parallels the growth of information policing functions, including regulating the flow of information nationally and internationally. Transnational policing is partly about the regulation of a new, growing and resonant kind of social space. Communicational policing, the ordering of 'cyberspace', is a growing facet of policing. The police role in formatting information exchange, monitoring the content, and reflecting these structures within the police organisation is of notable significance. Growth of a 'capacity' (an infrastructure of information technology) in policing is notable, even granted that it is largely potential and not actually present. This infrastructural capacity is unmistakably visible in the number of police forces using computer assisted dispatch, geo-coding for crime intelligence, mobile digital terminals and internet connections, as well as the growth of national (and transnational) police data-banks and dedicated computer networks. The development, in the UK, of a national crime faculty with links to the Home Office and a national criminal intelligence model, is but one example of what has been termed 'technology transfer' and its resultant circulations of knowledges (Sheptycki 1998d). While skill in using these tools is lacking, their development is ongoing and accelerating.

Terms such as 'intelligence-led' policing, popular in England and prominently featured as a strategic focus by the Kent County Constabulary, suggest that information is critical to the surveillance, monitoring, controlling and sanctioning of crime, including crimes with and by information processing devices. Thus, gathering and regulating information increasingly drives the growth of all forms of policing (see Sheptycki 2000). These functions can be called information policing, and refer to police capacity to gather intelligence (information in advance of a criminal incident), collate information as a result of detected crime, and to analytically store, retrieve and process this material (intelligence and information) relatively parsimoniously. To discover how information policing has emerged, it must be placed in the context of economic and social change.

In this chapter, I discuss the impact of several economic–communicational developments on policing and explore the hypothesis that the 'globalisation of policing', understood as territorially generalised and legitimate regulation of social processes, is now well under way. While policing remains an institutionalised means to apply force to protect and enhance governmental interests, the present situation requires re-imagining these interests. Transnational policing is regulation that extends between countries or, perhaps, from one country into another and this can happen both legally and illegally. It includes formal and informal joint surveillance efforts or criminal investigations that link police-type agencies from more than one nation. It also entails supranational groups such as UN peacekeeping forces, military–domestic linkages involving one nation's forces, and quasi-legal bodies such as Interpol. The emphasis on the active term found herein (that is, on policing, rather than on the police mandate) is intentional. Without analysis of dynamic policing transactions, one is left with stark formalism and typologies which are intellectually impoverished. Growth in the world economy, the decline in the power of the former Soviet Union and shifting conceptions of national interest, modes of regulation, and policing are the more salient changes that have shaped the current trend toward extra-territorial enforcement of laws and transnational policing. I explore transnational policing of information as a case in point.

Selected changes in the world economy

The growth of multinational corporations whose interests and subsidiary units extend globally, and whose loyalties are only nominally national, have obviated the simplistic identification of economic interests with state interests. The movement of cash and resources within these corporations has, according to some, 'emptied the state' because states' ability to control, tax and monitor monetary movements has diminished (see Sheptycki, this volume, chapter five). This decentralisation of state power and control is hotly dramatised by the decline and collapse of Russian power as a coherent economic–political force, as well as the dedifferentiation of several sovereign states out of the former Yugoslavia and states within the Soviet federation. Concomitantly, markets are both exploding and imploding. China is now the world's third largest economy and hosts some 10,000 named 'joint ventures', while Japan is 'downsizing' its indigenous manufacture of vehicles and shifting a larger proportion of its production to the United States and elsewhere (*Detroit Free Press*, 23 June 1996). Local practices and myriad trade rules exist in Eastern Europe and the former Soviet Union, and economic development both within and outwith the United States is uneven. Local control of markets by provinces and cities exists in China, in economic development zones within the United States and elsewhere.

At the same time, international trade practices and regulations are being affected by the existence of trade regimes such as the North American Free Trade Agreement (NAFTA), the European Union (EU), and the World Trade Organisation (WTO), while the United States' periodic designation of 'Preferred Nation' status to specific nations remains a contingent feature of global trade. These developments – particularly the work of the WTO – signal a movement toward centralisation and homogenisation of trade laws and practices and the growth of transnational politico-economic unions. It would do to note that, running counter to these trends is the creeping transnationalisation of the ecological crisis and rise of concepts of managed 'risk' rather than market forces as the principal underpinning of global relationships; witness the now world-wide 'Green Movement' and the anti-nuclear testing and anti-nuclear power movements in Europe (Beck 1992). The above noted changes in markets are complemented by the rise of contests over emerging 'market(s) in information' (Castells 1996). The notion that information is essential to strategic advantage, as I outline below, is becoming the new rhetoric of America's security establishment.

Changes in the nature of 'national interests'

The changing role of information in economics foreshadows the changes in its meaning and role in national security. Traditional economic thought held that information is slippery and often unavailable. Unlike a market in commodities or services, information was viewed as being capable only of being symbolically named, tracked, sold and bought. Information was an essential component of economic market stability. Friedrich August von Hayek and the Austrian School of economics, argued for interrelations of uncertainty and subjective assessments in (often unintended) market stability (von Hayek 1944/ 1994). In this view, genuine information is embedded in ignorance and endogenous forces, contingencies that are not fully predictable and understandable. The subjective side of market function means that disruptions and changes are enstructured by routines, rules and procedures that unintentionally stabilise complex markets and pattern them. This means, arguably, that the regulation of uncertain information markets will increasingly be both a cause and consequence of market dynamics. By developing enforcement procedures, regulators shape markets. The rules of thumb that enable best estimates of targeted behaviour create conditions under which information markets change. As the information monitoring infrastructure increases, the markets become reflexively tied into conceptions of the market, in turn based on modelling, simulation and computer-based controls on trading.

In the United States, the notion of the 'national interest', once based in 'anti-communism' reified in the guise of the Soviet Union, is necessarily being redefined. The United States government, in co-operation with large corporations, many in the defence industry, has broadened its definition of the national interest to include 'information' (read: industrial secrets and ideas with 'R and D' potential). Government and industry are now actively seeking to commodify information and to police its use and diffusion. Protected by linking military notions such as 'deterrence', 'domestic' or 'international intelligence', and 'counter-intelligence', the national interest now includes the security of information. While this includes the traditional classified and secret materials central to governing, the significance of the newly emergent view is that information security needs are now expanded to include strategic information useful for opening and maintaining markets, and for sustaining American economic, as well as military, suzerainty. Information held secure in the national interest entails both state-held and proprietary corporate information. This linguistic transformation of information as a basis for national strength and survival in the context of economic competition implies the obligation to use strategic means to protect and enhance it. Consequently extensions of strategy to assure the protection of information (waging a 'war', or an 'information war', and guarding diligently against external threats) are under way. Domestic security now includes diligent protection of information, intelligence-gathering and counter-intelligence to prevent industrial espionage (see the Introduction to this volume).

National interests are seen as vested in information as a property, product and process. The means by which information is created, analysed, processed, distributed, stored and exchanged is therefore 'strategic'. Such a view was preceded by the Industrial Security Initiative of the Bush Administration in 1992 which was reiterated in recent congressional testimony. The Director of the Central Intelligence Agency, John Deutsh, a former MIT Professor, testified before a Senate Subcommittee about the potential for disruptions in communications, threats to national interest due to potential loss of secrets, and for war(s) over information. According to him, an 'information war' could become a twenty-first-century national security threat second only to nuclear, biological and chemical weapons. *The New York Times* (Markoff 1996), coining a phrase, labelled these future contests 'cyberwars', a linguistic device upheld by Mr Deutsh who proposed creating a 'cyberwar center' in the National Security Agency.

Information is being redefined in legal terms as a form of property: intellectual property (Coombe 1998). Efforts to commodify information by transforming it into 'intellectual property', are indicated by the establishment of the National Information Property Law Center (at George Washington University); the current debate over photocopying rights (the demise of Kinko's course packets as a result of a suit by the publishing industry) and the growth of intellectual property offices in major research universities. These challenges are reshaping a legal doctrine in Anglo-American nations concerning the fine line between collective and individual interests in ownership of ideas via copyright laws dating to the late eighteenth century. According to Keith Aoki (1998), 'intellectual property rights cover too much and are still expanding, generating an intellectual property smog' (p. 274).[2] The transnational policing of intellectual property rights is problematic for at least two reasons. Firstly, intellectual property rights are private property rights, which has implications for freedom of speech (private parties do not engage in censorship, only governmental or public bodies do). Secondly, some types of intellectual property rights, for example those associated with 'bio-prospecting' (that is, patented genetic material), held by a few multinational companies, raise troubling international human rights and distributive issues (p. 260). The expanding scope of national and transnational intellectual property protection raises questions relevant to the sociology of policing that have not been addressed in that literature. To cite but one example, in October 1993 (on Mahatma Gandhi's birthday) half a million Indian farmers staged a mass protest at the Indian offices of Cargill Seeds Ltd (a subsidiary of the largest privately held corporation in the United States). They were protesting at what they saw as 'piracy by patent', since Cargill had patented a seed that had been used in their farming villages for centuries, with quite profound economic implications – positive ones for Cargill, negative ones for Indian farmers (pp. 273–4). Thus, Indian state police were brought in to control a public order situation arising out of conflict over the transnational assertion of intellectual property rights. We might therefore contend that the Indian state was aiding and abetting 'bio-piracy' against its own citizens.

The commodification of information is illustrated in a striking fashion by efforts to control access to, and use of, the internet. Commercialisation of exchanges on the internet is under way in spite of resistance by those who use it. Developed as a secure national defence network that would permit multiple links between computers in the event of war or other national crisis, the internet was then hived off to the National Science Foundation for support and development (Rheingold 1993: 7). Recent developments in the integration of control over access are indicated by the monopolistic practices of Microsoft and the consequent anti-trust suit pursued by the US Justice Department. These are aspects of the rapid commodification of the net and access to it. This potential for control lies behind the current competition in the US between telephone and cable television companies (being won by AT&T and others) for control over the use of fibre-optic cables. This suggests that future access to the internet may be controlled and billed by telephone companies as modems become obsolete. Attempts to regulate internet communication are being opened up using the wedge

of seeking to control 'cyberporn'. Further, and *a fortiori*, debates surrounding cryptography, the commercial v-chip, and other software
that blocks access and usage, suggest that regulation and control of
the world-wide web will not evolve on the model of 'free speech' or
'freedom of the press', but rather will unfold under the logic of commerce. In the United States this will be conceptualised as a form of
interstate commerce giving purview to the federal government. Clearly,
these centralisation trends are in conflict with the ideals of freedom of
speech and of the press. Crucially however, a June 1996 Federal District Court decision ruled that internet transactions are more akin to
free speech protected by the First Amendment than property exchange.

Unregulated flows of information and meta-information (such as
codes, software and encryption devices which reorganise data into
information, that is: data with social meaning) have always been threatening to commercial interests. The first signs of the computer revolution brought forth counter-efforts to control the distribution of software
(Critchley 1996). The invention of the PC and its later successful re-
finement and marketing by Apple, were driven initially by a democratic vision of spreading and diffusing mundane and technical
knowledge (programs). Microsoft changed that dramatically through
its control and marketing of the DOS system adopted by IBM. The
present movement to gain control of information via software and
marketing reproduces the successful attempt to control sales of software and restrict free access to large mainframe computers. A parallel
movement originating in Japan led to international monopolistic control by Nintendo and Sega of games components (Fallows 1994).

Competition exists within private industries and between private
industry and the US federal government. In addition to the Microsoft
anti-trust suit (only ambiguously resolved at the time of writing) other
attempts to crack the state-industrial monopoly on information exchange are seen in the form of illegal 'hacking' and computer piracy
(Shimomura and Markoff 1996). Not all break-ins are sinister in the
commercial sense, but some are intended to dramatise the struggle
for democratic control of information, and are part of the emerging
patterns of deviance and control on the net. The fantasy of complete
information control drives governmental concern for security. This is
so especially because the villains, the security system and the data are
in cyberspace and information can be stolen, copied, shifted about,
and used without leaving any obvious traces of mischief. In 1996 the
US Government Accounting Office reported that 250,000 hackers had
penetrated Department of Defense (DoD) computers and were 60 per
cent successful (US GAO 1996). An ironic twist to this is that corpora-

tions who use encryption (passwords based on the factoring of prime numbers) as protection against random penetration and industrial espionage, are being courted by software corporations who announce in the media when they have been able to break into 'secure systems'. They do this to demonstrate that corporations are vulnerable and should purchase the protection they are selling! (Robinson 1999). Thus, the premodern predations of Jonathan Wild are re-enacted in the contemporary efforts of private police-type agents who would offer 'security' to private corporations' cyberspace.

Corporations are now concerned about protection of industrial secrets that notionally constitute their competitive advantage in world markets. Economic espionage is perceived as a major threat and some 54 nations have been identified as engaged in economic espionage (DeGenaro 1996). This is not a simple problem because global corporations operate in many legal contexts, and are governed completely by none. Some nations, such as The People's Republic of China, do not respect international copyright agreements. What is commercially acceptable to sell and trade internationally may be, and usually is, inconsistent with US governmental designations of classified information. Conversely, what may be traded abroad without protection or recourse to government intervention may be viewed by a corporation as its core secrets. Some corporations, 3M for example, have detailed corporate policy on espionage and counter-intelligence activities which sets a higher standard than many governments would use in framing their practices of intelligence gathering and counter-intelligence. On the other hand, some corporations, such as computer software manufacturers who develop guidance systems for aircraft and missiles, are eager to trade in international markets but are prohibited from full participation because of US government policy and security interests made concrete in the form of official sanctions against selected countries. The interests of corporations and governments are frequently inconsistent.

This redefinition of national interests and the role of federal agencies in their protection has wide-ranging ramifications reflective of other trends: the dedifferentiation of national interests and territories, and changes in informal social control based on wide distribution of access to information technology and the mass media (especially television).

Changes in the locus of control

The growth of information policing as an orchestrated practice is not unrelated to the decline in other modes of social control and so a review of these, with specific reference to developments in the United States, is relevant. Consider social interaction between persons, once face-to-face, that are now mediated by an information-processing device. It should be noted that access to information channels, particularly the internet and other forms of computing power, is patterned by ethnicity, class, age and education, and that the costs of access and use are a form of stratification. This sociological generalisation holds true across the variety of industrial powers. Citizens in developing countries not only lack access, but these nations are dependent on developed countries' manufacturing parts, creating networks, installing satellite systems, and maintaining extant facilities (Castells 1996). Traditionally, self-control, whether understood to be provided by the super-ego, the me, the significant other, or through primary group processes, has been considered the foundational source of social control. These early twentieth-century formulations, by George Herbert Mead (1936) and fellow pragmatists, assumed face-to-face interaction, co-presence, wherein the myriad of cues given and given off are assessed directly. Increasingly, interpersonal processes are mediated and produced by the mass media and aspects of modern experience are derived from electronically represented images rather than exclusively from direct, sensate personal experience (Poster 1990). The interposition of visual media alters the relationship between an audience, performance and self so that expressive performance, once bound by mutually shared expressive burdens, becomes less constrained. New social realities (definitions of the real and the significant) are framed by media, and by computer screens which create ersatz social realities.

Extensive and powerful mediated interactions now may shape organisational as well as personal life, and even compete with face-to-face experiences for salience. Computers with screens enabling various forms of visual interaction, whether in the form of 'surfing' the worldwide web, playing video games, or participating in bulletin boards, FACs, MUDs, or other interactive sites, permit interactions to exist stripped free of specific settings, times, people or places (Meyrowitz 1985; Gergen 1991). Furthermore, this interaction can be carried out with code-words, passwords, false or notional identities, or with no direct connection to a social role (identified by a work, family, or personal attribute) (cf. Mann and Sutton 1998). Skilled users can masquerade via false names, codes, origins of their messages and deceptive programs (Shimomura and Markoff 1996). The internet is a visual text that displays and distributes dreams, fantasies, fears and passions as well as information narrowly conceived. It is increasingly difficult to distinguish and mark the limits of these electronic realities or predict

how they will shape interactional vicissitudes. The self is a highly problematic source of social control in this context.

New 'artificial selves' are created by means of 'bots' or software that
profiles types of consumers and typifies individual users. Amazon.com,
for example, has a program called 'Eyes' that will watch out for books,
records, or other consumables that fit your tastes as profiled by previously conducted queries. 'Cookies', or caches of files surfed, can be
monitored and used for market research. It is now possible for parents
to buy software to block access of users (their children) to certain sites
or sites with key words (e.g. sexual in nature), thus providing a techno-
mechanical surrogate for actual monitoring and control by adults
(Myers 1999). Similar mechanisms are being marketed for encrypting
messages on the internet or for increasing governmental controls over
security-sensitive information through encryption. Within the internet,
new forms of controls are emerging which substitute mechanical-
electronic means for interpersonal social controls; these include site
access fees, licensing fees for use of certain software and fees for access
analogous to pay-for-view cable television channels.

On the other hand, electronically mediated relations, organised
around e-mail, the world-wide web, pagers, cellular phones, and fax
machines, create, enhance, sustain and destroy relationships, and forge
links between otherwise distant and unconnected people (Gergen 1991;
Rheingold 1993). These relations range from quite intimate relations,
such as courtship and 'cyber-sex', via chat-rooms, trading of erotic
pictures, sounds and texts, to business transactions. Indeed, human
play is being reconfigured by cyber-technology; 'surfing', following
one's curiosity across sites, hearing messages, watching videos, reading
texts, or seeing amazing graphic displays, is a matter of routine for
younger people, if not for their mature counterparts. In the contemporary period the daily newspapers contain many stories of people who
find love and friendship, or are raped, defrauded and otherwise compromised as a result of internet-based interactions. In extreme cases
death (most often of the existential, as opposed to virtual, sort) may
be the result of such mediated communication. Informal modes of
control have arisen in these virtual spaces as well. In the 'virtual social
space' created by list-servers, on-line chat-rooms, and other virtual
communities verbally beating people up (known as 'flaming'), banish-
ment and gossip, all play such a role.

Claims have emerged that web surfing is addictive, that it is a neu-
rosis that destroys families and other traditional social ties. Our understanding of these changes in interpersonal relations (which is partially
shaped by mass media accounts) affects manners, customs and etiquette,

as well as selves. Unlike the 'collective consciousness' (Durkheim 1961) that links concrete interactions through practices with norms and values, modern media and information technology frame one sort of reality which is at once set apart from everyday life and yet is an intimate part of it. This is productive of multiple and, to an extent, arbitrarily connected social realities laminated in a stylised fashion and governed by media logic rather than grand integrating notions like religion or nationalism. Tensions exist in framing meaning because meanings can be located in various social realities, and easily changed by reframing them, for example, by turning a serious message into an ironic one, a news story into a film, a sporting competition into a spectacle, and looping media images playfully and cynically into new contexts (Manning 1996a, 1996b).

Legal controls have thus far been unevenly applied to the internet. Although there have been high-profile cases where police officers have themselves posed as paedophiles in order to entice others into illegalities (such as using the mail or telephones to dispense goods), and occasionally an arrest is made as a result (Wall 1998), more conventional forms of crime committed using computers (such as fraud, embezzlement, and money laundering) are not well-monitored by police forces, municipal, national or transnational because, in general, police lack the knowledge and expertise to investigate such crimes. The publicity and dramaturgy occasioned by the rare capture of 'hackers' indicates the paucity of actual surveillance and sanctioning (Shimomura and Markoff 1996). This is probably only a temporary state of affairs. The computer industry and universities have combined to develop Alert Centers, most notably the one at Carnegie-Mellon in Pittsburgh, that monitor and spread information to users about 'hackers', breaks in security, threatening viruses and new protections against computer system penetration. Such Alert Centers form the hub of a new form of policing in the information age and their reach will, of necessity, be transnational.

An emerging area that has yet to be fully exploited as a source of deviance and control by information police is that of surveillance and simulation in various combinations (Bogard 1996). Included here are several new modes of gathering information internationally. Private corporations have a vast dataveillance capacity which allows them to monitor many information transactions, aggregate them and create lists for marketing purposes, internal surveillance or evaluation and this has profound implications for the institution of privacy. George Ritzer (1995) has discussed the threat to privacy in the 'credit card society' (pp. 115–23) wherein he noted a plan hatched in 1990 by

Equifax and Lotus Development Corporation which was only aborted because of public uproar. Baldly, the plan was to market a CD-ROM containing information on about 150 million people including their names, addresses, approximate income, personal buying habits, and other lifestyle, demographic and income information. Such information remains available to big retailers, banks and other credit organisations, but the 1990 effort would have made it available to anyone with a computer. Ritzer quoted the editor of *Privacy Times*, to the effect that 'once they have established this precedent, there is nothing to stop the next guy from selling anything he wants [for use on a personal computer] from your Christmas purchases to your genetic history' (p. 115). While it still remains the case that these massive databases are not available to just anyone, such data are accessible to a number of institutions, most notably the credit industry, banks and the government. Quoting the former chairman of the US Privacy Protection Commission, Ritzer reinforced the point that 'the danger is that employers, banks and government agencies will use data bases to make decisions about our lives without our knowing about it' (p. 122). While the police have long had the co-operation of credit card companies in pursuing fraud and criminals using credit cards, the security system now has devised ways to profile those at risk of 'credit card abuse'. The notion of profiling and typifying gained notoriety during a controversy that emerged in the United States in the 1990s about the racial overtones of 'crime profiling'. Such techniques use simulations of characteristics to produce stereotypes of likely violators of drug, immigration, or traffic laws (Goldberg 1999). Once large networks of information are linked, profiles can be created of offenders and other suspect populations and applied to the public at large. Surveillance of everyday activity by monitoring credit card purchases for the use of parking lots, supermarket purchases, catalogue shopping and the like generates data that can in turn be used to profile, model and anticipate behaviour.

Nor is electronic surveillance limited to tracking footprints in cyberspace. Satellite pictures of great clarity and resolution, able to detect objects as small as one metre, can now be purchased by corporations or individuals. These images are limited by licence or by *ad hoc* 'shutter control' over certain satellites (Editorial, *New York Times* 1999). The growth in formal control mechanisms is complemented by a reduction in consensus and informal social control, and an accompanying movement towards 'cyber-control'. This is evident in the massive visual simulation of control witnessed in the first fully televised 'war as spectacle': the Gulf War (Kellner 1992). The bombing of Kosovo also relied on virtual command and control, satellite pictures rather than on-site observations (Ignatieff 1999). Electronic information technology alters the nature of informal social control (Zuboff 1988; Manning 1996a, 1996b), and changes the character of formal governmental social control. It raises the question of the fragile nature of information markets and their vulnerabilities.

Changes in policing

In this section I am interested primarily in information policing, or the use of information by third parties to control grievances. Formal modes of control are inversely related to informal modes, and the dance is one of expansion and contraction rather than ever-escalating formal powers (Black 1996). A number of trends in social control that shape information policing, arise in part from the above listed changes in social organisation and markets.

The first trend is the growth of transnational and quasi-legal police organisations (Benyon et al. 1993; Fijnaut 1993; Nadelmann 1993). This has been well-reviewed elsewhere in this book and need not detain us here. A second, perhaps more worrying, trend is periodic expansion of the willingness of the United States to enforce its laws extra-territorially and unilaterally. Begun in war and stimulated by terrorism and pan-national movements, the United States has extended domestic 'drug wars' by using military troops as well as DEA and FBI agents abroad. Nadelmann (1993) has documented this extensively. At this point, we can note that in May 1996 the US Government Accounting Office announced a decline in American efforts in the Caribbean and, further, that it regularly reported the failure of virtually every operation of this kind over the previous decade. The Ker-Frisbie doctrine in US law is clear evidence of the US predilection for extra-territorial law enforcement beyond the bounds of both treaty and customary law. This doctrine is especially evident in the case of US v. Alvarez-Machain. In this case a Mexican citizen who was alleged to have assisted in the kidnapping and killing of a DEA agent in Mexico, was forcibly abducted in Mexico and brought to trial in the United States. The US Supreme Court upheld the conviction of Alvarez-Machain, ruling that this mode of bringing him to trial (stuffing him into the boot of a car and smuggling him across the border secretly) did not constitute a due process violation. This conviction was later overturned on appeal on other grounds. These interventions are paralleled by the international use of force which is sometimes, but not always, internationally sanctioned, if only by a few nations (loyal allies).

A third trend is the growth of the power of transnational policing through mutual assistance and multinational agreements such as Mutual Legal Assistance Treaties (MLATs) and Memoranda of Understanding (MoUs). Additionally, according to a number of authors it appears that US police tactics are being diffused into countries which had not known them previously. These include various undercover methods associated with the 'war on drugs', not least of which is the popular practice of 'controlled delivery' (Nadelmann 1993; Fijnaut and Marx 1995; Sheptycki 1996). What appears to be happening is that transnational agreements for mutual assistance between law enforcement agencies are being ironed out in the wake of police operations both successful and otherwise, that is: police practice sets the frame for legal regulation, rather than vice versa.

A fourth and significant trend which has, thus far, gone largely unexplored in the literature is expansion into industrial espionage by the FBI, DEA, NSA and CIA which is concomitant with the end of the Cold War and attendant 'high police' functions (Brodeur 1983). This extension serves to reshape the police mandate; to focus it and engage in 'cyber' or information wars. The now accepted idea that information occupies a space, cyberspace, and that this imaginary world is subject to policing and control is an important epistemological and metaphysical shift. Symbolic space is now as open to policing as physically defined space. The *New York Times* (4 September 1999) reported that the Justice Department is proposing legislation that would allow agents to enter homes and disable any encryption devices the residents owned, and/or install devices that would allow them to 'read' or decode an encrypted text. The Federal Communications Commission, at the urging of the Justice Department, has adopted new rules concerning monitoring of cellular phone calls and callers – now over 55 million subscribers in the US (Fleming 1999) – allowing tracking of movements of users (by call location, on the basis of a warrant) through the phone companies. A literature on computer crime is growing and the FBI is vigorously recruiting new agents with computer skills. It is widely known that the FBI monitored internet transactions carried out by the 'Freemen' while barricaded inside their isolated ranch during the Siege of Montana in 1997. Less well known is the fact that the FBI now has a specialised unit for 'economic espionage' (headed by Kenneth Geide) which actively seeks industry co-operation in identifying information loss and other economic crimes. Perhaps not surprisingly, the CIA intends to monitor international economic crimes and to protect information, if the Director's congressional testimony in 1996 is an indication.

Comments and conclusions

Several paradoxes remain to be dramatised. While there is evidence of formal and informal co-operation among police-type agencies both nationally and transnationally, it is also clear that much conflict and competition also exists (Sheptycki 1998c). Competition between agencies is apparent within the United States and Europe and, again, this is true of co-operation both within and across the various states. While something is known of the form of co-operative relationships, little is known of the actual 'content' of information exchanged between agencies and the consequences, if any, of such exchanges. This remains difficult to determine for any given force, let alone international exchanges, and yet this is likely to hold the key to understanding the emergent transnational police 'system'. An increase in the frequency and number of queries to the National Criminal Intelligence Center (NCIC) or Interpol, for example, replicates the police concern with the means of policing, rather than the ends, with process rather than outcomes. In 1994, the FBI purchased a new, vast, computer system (Sarbin 1997) because the validity of the data the NCIC computer contained was dubious, and few controls had been exercised in accepting or erasing warrant information. Similar observations have been made about Interpol databases (Sheptycki 1995). This suggests that the view of Ericson and Haggerty (1997) that police are 'information workers', based on formal ties and networks, is somewhat problematic, in part because the argument refers to potential and form, rather than content and actual use. Extended accessible information networks, such as that connected to the FBI's fingerprint databank, will alter practice (Walsh 1999), as will standardised radio links within vast metropolitan areas such as Dallas-Fort Worth. And yet, the argument for unification via communicational networks overlooks the vapid, unreliable and invalid content of much of the information present within policing data archives (Geller and Morris 1992). Moreover, the lack of systematic use of computer-based information as well as police resistance to the application of new analytic tools associated with such information (or inability to use them) are just as likely to shape the contours of the emerging system.

Changes in the nature of external threats to governments are seen in the rhetoric of 'information security' and the 'information war' in the United States. These are variations on the threat of the drug cartels and previously of the Soviet Union and communism. The character of the posited external other, the 'folk devils' (Cohen 1972), does not appear uniform internationally. Terrorism, drug markets and illegal immigration particularly have been used to justify much police co-operation and joint operations in Europe and some of the pressure for such co-operation even originates at the ministerial level (Anderson et al. 1995; Sheptycki 1996). While the international agreements, *ad hoc* policing taskforces, and semi-permanent policing groups that are grow-ing in number across Europe do so with reference to these particular folk devils (Sheptycki 1995), by comparison the United States' con-cerns remain chauvinistic, driven as much by economic and informa-tion-security concerns (Marenin 1998). These are echoed and amplified in efforts to extend the laws of the United States extra-territorially. In the contemporary period, North American criminologists are studying facets of the international spread of crime, in particular Russian and Asian 'organized crime groups', gang activity, Colombian drug car-tels, drug trafficking, and economic espionage (Shelley 1990). It seems clear that the collapse of the Soviet Union has produced symbolic dysplasia.

'Computer crime' remains an undefined sink into which many con-flicting ideas are poured. The most urgent threats, targets of control and villainous enemies are unclear. Many are symbolic or exist in cyberspace. The putative internal enemies remain and the cyberpunks are simply additions to the already established lexicon of folk devilry: illegal immigrants, and those who smuggle them, people of colour generally and particularly African-American youths, anti-government populist anarchists (the 'Freemen' and other rural radicals), as well as white youths influenced by video games, media violence, and insecure school environments. Illicit drugs remain a mysterious and evil threat which, all too often, is erroneously drawn in popular discourse as exclusively the problem of the lower classes, a problem that requires tough criminal sanctions and no more. Meanwhile, drug use in the higher echelons – say, for example, in Beverly Hills or Manhattan – remains much less visible (and hence less subject to criminal sanction) and licit drugs and patent medicines such as tobacco, alcohol, Prozac and Viagra are regulated via civil law. The distortions in social control priorities that emanate from the predilection to 'wage war on drugs' may well come to affect policing in the new social spaces in unpredict-able ways. What is also true is that the war on drugs gains powerful new tools by virtue of the capacity of policing-type agencies to patrol virtual reality.

The growth of internationalism in enforcement has largely been defined formally, with reference to legality (Benyon et al. 1993; Sheptycki 1995) and, indeed, 'topologically'. This growth has been paralleled by the rise of networks of chaos and terror, and alternatives to state-based governance and transnational movements. Consider the growth of sea and air piracy; terrorism; the huge network of private policing which has transnational linkages (see Johnston this volume); and pan-national liberation groups (for example, Hezbollah). These compete for the monopoly of force, and put the lie to the Weberian theme of monopoly of violence as a key defining feature of state policing. Rapid and cheap transportation, miniature explosive devices, free movement within the EU, and transnational corporate movements of information, especially electronic fund transfers, constrain enforcement, whether based on 'national interests' or redefined as international threats. The laws of Western countries and, indeed, the legal canopy in many developing countries (which is, in many instances, based on European law), reflect nineteenth-century ideas concerning privacy, institutional insulation from public law, deterrence, the 'rational man', and property. Cyberspace is a new social space that can only be defined analogously and metaphorically. The information networks that comprise this new environment are altering these nineteenth-century ideas. Information-based policing moves away from the founding notions of policing based on the idea of benign reaction to public nuisance, crime and control of riots or disorder. Based on surveillance and simulation (modelling of the future based on present data), and abetted by means to monitor information networks, policing will increasingly encompass notions of intervention and prevention, intelligence-gathering and analysis, counter-intelligence and disinformation, largely based on electronically gathered, stored, processed and transmitted information. We are as yet unable to predict the direction and consequences of 'the net' (Rochlin 1998). Because the processes of control work analogically and metaphorically rather than literally, the representations of transnational crimes are increasingly important. The growth of the fears and risks of cybercrime are a product of several non-independent forces. The 'watchdogs', heads of security at computer and telephone corporations (a misleading distinction), are themselves working at the emerging edges of legality and ethics by breaking into corporate records, demonising a few individuals while stripping them of moral credibility, all the while exaggerating the costs and risks of 'hacking' through inflated statements about the associated losses, to elevate their own status while breaking the law themselves (Goodell 1996). This enterprise, a form of moral entrepreneurship, is driven also by the complicity and active involvement of media figures in the investigations, publicity, alerts and panics surrounding computer 'break-ins' (Shimomura and Markoff 1996). The language of cybercrime refers to physical, not virtual, realities. It treats information as property that can be 'secure', 'violated', 'compromised', 'stolen' or 'valued' in monetary terms. It introduces trust and contractual obligations as a basis for electronic transactions, and personalises data files. These linguistic turns are in turn amplified by the contextual work of the media which elevates fears and pressures for national and world-wide enforcement. In short, policing in new social spaces has produced new, ever more shrill, claims for crime-threat control by police (both public and private) and has stimulated new rhetorical devices, presentational strategies and innovative organisational tactics that are helping to reshape policing in the twenty-first century.

Notes

1 A version of this paper was presented at the meetings of the Law and Society Association, Strathclyde University, Glasgow, Scotland, 10–13 July 1996.
2 Since June 1996, five bills have been introduced in Congress intending to provide coherent protection of the economic secrets of the United States. Two of the five contain provisions for the enforcement of American commercial law abroad to protect information.

References

Anderson, M. (1989) *Policing the World*, Oxford: Clarendon Press.
Anderson, M., den Boer, M., Cullen, P., Gilmore, W., Raab, C., and Walker, N. (1995) *Policing the European Union: Theory, Law and Practice*, Oxford: Clarendon Press.
Aoki, K. (1998) 'The Stakes of Intellectual Property Law', in D. Kairys (ed.), *The Politics of Law: A Progressive Critique*, 3rd edition, New York: Basic Books.
Bayley, D. (1975) 'The Police and Political Development in Europe', in C. Tilley (ed.), *The Formation of National States in Europe*, Princeton NJ: Princeton University Press.
Beck, U. (1992) *Risk Society: Toward a New Modernity*, London: Sage.
Benyon, J., Turnbull, L., Willis, A., Woodward, R. and Beck, A. (1993) *Police Co-operation in Europe: An Investigation*, Leicester: Centre for the Study of Public Order, University of Leicester.
Bittner, E. (1970) *The Functions of the Police in Modern Society*, Chevy Chase MD: National Institute of Mental Health.
Black, D. (1996) *The Social Structure of Right and Wrong*, New York: Academic Press.
Bogard, W. (1996) *The Simulation of Surveillance*, Cambridge: Cambridge University Press.
Bourdieu, P. (1977) *Outline of a Theory of Practice*, Cambridge: Cambridge University Press.

Brewer, J. D., Guelke, A., Hume, I., Moxon-Browne, E., and Wilford, R. (1988) *The Police, Public Order and the State*, New York: St. Martin's.

Brodeur, J.-P. (1983) 'High Policing and Low Policing: Remarks about the Policing of Political Activities', *Social Problems*, Vol. 30, No. 5, pp. 507–20.

Brogden, M. and Shearing, C. (1993) *Policing for a New South Africa*, London: Routledge.

Castells, M. (1996) *The Rise of the Network Society*, Oxford: Blackwell.

Cohen, S. (1972) *Folk Devils and Moral Panics*, London: Paladin.

Cohen, S. (1995) 'State Crimes of Previous Regimes: Knowledge, Acountability and the Policing of the Past', *Law and Social Inquiry: Journal of the American Bar Foundation*, Vol. 20, No. 1, pp. 7–50.

Cohen, S. (1996) 'Government Responses to Human Rights Reports: Claims, Denials and Counter Claims', *Human Rights Quarterly*, Vol. 18, No. 3, pp. 517–43.

Coombe, R. (1998) *The Cultural Life of Intellectual Properties*, Durham NC: Duke University Press.

Critchley, R. (1996) *Accidental Empires: How the Boys of Silicon Valley Make Their Millions, Battle Foreign Competition and Still Can't Get a Date*, Reading MA: Addison-Wesley.

DeGenaro, W. (1996) 'Security and Counter-intelligence', unpublished paper presented to The Seminar on Security, Michigan State University, May.

Detroit Free Press (1996) 'Japan Increasing US Production', 23 June.

Durkheim, E. (1961) *Elementary Forms of the Religious Life*, New York: Collier Books.

Ericson, R. and Haggerty, K. (1997) *Policing the Risk Society*, Toronto: University of Toronto Press.

Fallows, J. (1994) 'The Computer Wars' *New York Review of Books*, 24 March.

Fijnaut, C. (ed.) (1993) *The Internationalization of Police Co-operation in Western Europe*, Deventer: Kluwer.

Fijnaut, C. and Marx, G. (1995) *Undercover: Police Surveillance in Comparative Perspective*, The Hague: Kluwer.

Fleming, A. T. (1999) 'Cell Phone Leaves Society Disconnected' *Lansing State Journal*, 14 August.

Gall, C. (1999) 'Community Policing Taught by Americans in Kosovo', *New York Times*, 8 September 1999.

Geller, W. and Morris, N. (1992) 'Relations between Federal and Local Police', in M. Tonry and N. Morris (eds), *Modern Policing*, Chicago: University of Chicago Press.

Gergen, K. (1991) *The Saturated Self: Dilemmas of Identity in Contemporary Life*, New York: Basic Books.

Giddens, A. (1991) *Modernity and Self-Identity*, Cambridge: Polity Press.

Goldberg, J. (1999) 'The Color of Suspicion', *New York Times Magazine*, 20 June.

Goodell, J. (1996) *The Cyberthief and the Samurai*, New York: Dell.

Haggerty, K. and Ericson, R. V. (1999) 'The Militarization of Policing in the Information Age', *Journal of Political and Military Sociology*, Vol. 27 (Winter), pp. 233–55.

Harding, C., Fennell, P., Jörg, N. and Swart, B. (eds) (1995) *Criminal Justice in Europe: A Comparative Study*, Oxford: Clarendon Press.

Hayek, F. A. von (1944/1994) *The Road to Serfdom*, Chicago: University of Chicago Press.

Ignatieff, M. (1999) 'The Virtual Commander', *The New Yorker*, 2 August, pp. 30–6.

Kraska, P. and Kappeler, V. (1997) 'Militarizing American Police', *Social Problems*, Vol. 44, pp. 1–18.

Kellner, D. (1992) *The Persian Gulf TV War*, Boulder CO: Westview.

Lee, J. (1999) 'Capturing No-so-still Life: Beams in Many Flavours', *New York Times*, 2 September.

Mann, D. and Sutton, M. (1998) 'NETCRIME: More Change in the Organization of Thieving', *British Journal of Criminology*, Vol. 38, No. 2, pp. 201–29.

Manning, P. K. (1996a) 'Media Loops', in F. Bailey and D. Hale (eds), *Media, Culture and Crime*, Belmont: Wadsworth.

Manning, P. K. (1996b) 'Dramaturgy, Politics and the Axial Media Event', *Sociological Quarterly*, Vol. 37, pp. 101–18.

Marenin, O. (1998) 'United States Police Assistance to Emerging Democracies', *Policing and Society*, Vol. 8, No. 2, pp. 153–68.

Markoff, J. (1996) 'Cyberwars Coming', *New York Times*, 26 June.

Mead G. H. (1936) *Mind, Self and Society*, Charles Morris (ed.), Chicago: University of Chicago Press.

Meyrowitz, J. (1985) *No Sense of Place: The Impact of Electronic Media on Social Behaviour*, New York: Oxford University Press.

Myers, M. (1999) 'Softeyes Tracks Kids' Web Visits', *Lansing State Journal*, 24 August.

Nadelmann, E. (1993) *Cops Across Borders: The Internationalization of US Criminal Law Enforcement*, University Park, PA: Pennsylvania State University Press.

New York Times (1999) 'Intrusions on Electronic Privacy', Editorial, 4 September 1999.

Poster, M. (1990) *The Mode of Information*, Chicago: University of Chicago Press.

Rheingold, H. (1993) *Virtual Reality*, New York: HarperCollins.

Rheinstein, M. (1954/1969) *Max Weber on Law in Economy and Society*, Cambridge MA: Harvard University Press.

Ritzer, G. (1995) *Expressing America: A Critique of the Global Credit Card Society*, Thousand Oaks CA: Pine Forge Press.

Robinson, S. (1999) 'Internet Code-cracking Project Shows Need for Stronger Locks', *New York Times*, 6 September.

Rochlin, E. (1998) *Caught in the Net*, Princeton NJ: Princeton University Press.

Sarbin, T. (ed.) (1997) *Vision 2021: Security Issues for the Next Quarter Century*, Monterey CA: Defense Security Research Center.

Shelley, L. (1990) 'The Internationalization of Crime: The Changing Relationship between Crime and Development', pp. 119–34 in U. Zvekic (ed.), *Essays on Crime and Development*, Rome: UN Interregional Crime and Justice Research Institute.

Sheptycki, J. (1995) 'Transnational Policing and the Makings of a Postmodern State', *British Journal of Criminology*, Vol. 35, No. 4, pp. 613–35.

Sheptycki, J. (1996) 'Law Enforcement, Justice and Democracy in the Transnational Arena: Reflections on the War on Drugs', *International Journal of the Sociology of Law*, Vol. 24, No. 1, pp. 61–75.

Sheptycki, J. (1997) 'Transnationalism, Crime Control and the European State System: A Review of the Literature', *International Criminal Justice Review*, Vol. 7, pp. 130–40.

Sheptycki, J. (1998a) 'The Global Cops Cometh: Reflections on Transnationalization, Knowledge Work and Policing Subculture', *British Journal of Sociology*, Vol. 49, No. 1, pp. 57–74.

Sheptycki, J. (1998b) 'Policing, Postmodernism and Transnationalisation', *British Journal of Criminology*, Vol. 38, No. 3, pp. 485–503.

Sheptycki, J. W. E. (1998c) 'Police Co-operation in the English Channel Region, 1968–1996', *European Journal of Crime, Criminal Law and Criminal Justice*, Vol. 6, No. 3, pp. 216–35.

Sheptycki, J. W. E. (1998d) 'Reflections on the Transnationalisation of Policing: The Case of the RCMP and Serial Killers', *International Journal of the Sociology of Law*, Vol. 26, pp. 17–34.

Sheptycki, J. W. E. (ed.) (2000) *Intelligence-led Policing: A Policing and Society Special Issue*, Vol. 9, No. 4, pp. 311–14.

Shimomura, T. and Markoff, J. (1996) *Takedown*, New York: Hyperion Books.

US GAO (1996) 'Computer Hackers Penetrate Defence Computers', *GAO Report*, June.

Wall, D. (1998) 'Catching Cybercriminals: Policing the internet', *International Review of Law, Computers and Technology*, Vol. 12, No. 2, pp. 201–18.

Walsh, E. (1999) 'FBI Lops Time Off Fingerprint Checks', *Lansing State Journal*, 10 September.

Wright, R. (1999) 'Private Eyes', *New York Times Magazine*, 5 May.

Zuboff, S. (1988) *In the Age of the Smart Machine*, New York: Basic Books.

7 The 'drug war'

Learning from the paradigm example of transnational policing

James Sheptycki

Introduction

While the evolution of the transnational state system is ongoing, theories of globalisation remain partial and contingent. Perhaps adequate theorisation of the 'new world order' awaits the benefit of historical hindsight. However, the practical concerns of active researchers are not the handmaidens of already established theories. Rather, social scientific research, like normal science in general, is more often the unreflective application of disciplinary technique. Political scientists, sociologists, geographers, socio-legalists, economists and others have already embarked on the business of describing, analysing and prescribing the practices that make up the transnational order. In doing so they have, perhaps without noticing it, begun to come to terms with the policing practices that patrol the conduct of the global system. Criminologists, whose disciplinary focus is limited, in some cases with reluctance, to the concerns of the criminal law, have tended to look only at those aspects of policing that pertain to law enforcement. But, as indicated at the outset of this volume, policing is not mere law enforcement and a full account of its transnational aspects or, indeed, policing in a purely national context, should not be so limited. Policing is a crucial building block of governance. As such, the study of transnational policing offers a window onto the emerging governmental practices of the transnational state system and this is why, when it is considered in its broadest sense, policing is of interest to many outside the narrow world of criminology. The contributions to this book show something of the potential of this broader research agenda. They indicate that many disciplinary discourses can be exercised by the questions that arise. It should therefore be apparent to the reader that there is, as yet, an unfulfilled research agenda on issues relating to transnational policing.

However, there is no escaping the fact that much of the research concerning transnational policing has, thus far, remained within a narrow ambit. That is why, upon explaining to casual acquaintances and colleagues that one is engaged in studying transnational policing, the invariable response is: 'Oh, so you are studying drug trafficking'. Crimes associated with the illicit market in psychoactive substances have underwritten much of the public understanding of the need to foster the transnational police enterprise. This is an understandable state of affairs. International agreements have constrained and shaped national policies in the drugs field for virtually the entire twentieth century, making drug policy the flagship of transnational law enforcement. The implications of this for the shaping of the transnational state system are quite profound, and this is likely to have special interest for political scientists and those interested in international law, since some of these international agreements adopted notions of 'universal applicability' (Joint Study Group 1980).[1] Universal applicability means that those countries acceding to (and/or signing, and/or ratifying – whatever the formal requirements happen to be) international agreements are prepared to force countries that have not done so to obey nonetheless or to face censure, in the form of trade embargoes and other sanctions. This means that pursuit of global drug prohibition has had important implications for *the* basic element of the system of international law, namely the concept of state sovereignty. Any new function that is ascribed as a transnational police enterprise in the twenty-first century will also probably require such a licence. It is thus worth considering the history of international drug controls, even if only in outline form. This is not simply because drug prohibition dominates the contemporary agenda for research on transnational policing but, even more prosaically, because its evolution over the course of the twentieth century tells us so much about the transnational system.[2]

Challenging the functional assumptions of international drug prohibition

It is common to describe the international agenda that relates to drugs in relation to its proclaimed functional aims. It is difficult to take issue with those who presuppose that policy-makers declared the so-called 'drug war' in order to preserve the health of societies in which it has been waged. Historically, drug use has been depicted in the mass media as something likely to destroy the very foundations of the social order. Since the menace is so plain, the reasoning goes, the control efforts must be ruthless (Cloyd 1982). Using just this rationale it was possible for President George Bush to reaffirm the United States' commitment to the drug war, calling for more police, more prisons and stiffer penalties for traffickers and consumers alike (Grazia 1991). He was even able to call for more participation of the American military and state security apparatus in the prosecution of the drug war at roughly the same time as revelations emerged from the Iran-Contra inquiry which implicated quite senior personnel from those very institutions in international drug trafficking. That he could do so without apology and without a trace of irony is testimony to the strength of the functional rationale, not to say rhetoric, of the social response to drug use and the entrenched logic of drug prohibition. In the context of pronounced worries about the extent of the drug problem in the early 1990s it proved impossible for the newly elected president Bill Clinton to act on the impulse to rationalise the drug law enforcement apparatus by merging several of the federal agencies concerned with this effort. Representatives of the DEA, in particular, were vociferous in promoting the view that the extent of the drug problem was such that the US government required extensive and multiple agencies in order to successfully wage a war against it. When William Bennett, the Director of the Office of Drug Control Policy in the USA, stated in 1989 that 'drugs represent the gravest present threat to our national well-being' because 'our drug problem is getting worse', he did so after decades of the drug war (quoted in Zimring and Hawkins 1997: 5). His response was to call for an intensification of previous practice, that is: more enforcement. Some have attempted to argue that the emphasis on prohibition advocated under official ODCP policy produces unacceptable 'collateral damage', including the exacerbation of drug-related crime, the deepening of racial and class divisions, the undermining of treatment and prevention measures and a concomitant exacerbation of health risks (Bertram et al. 1996). Others have suggested that, apart from the negative consequences that stem from the neglect of the public health dimensions, the emphasis on drug law *enforcement* fosters 'the potential exploitation of the drug problem as a rallying point for authoritarian sentiments in American society' (Zimring and Hawkins 1997: 21). That the cure of a social ill like drug abuse might be iatrogenic is cause for concern. That the prescriptions of drug prohibition continue to be followed in spite of manifest failure is, perhaps, the most compelling reason to discard the functional rationale that is used to explain its deployment.

Our understanding of these matters is clarified when we look at the drug prohibition outside of parameters pertaining to national policies for the control of drug use (for example Bean 1974; Wilson 1985: 195–

222) and instead examine it in the context of the evolving transnational state system during the twentieth century. It is indisputable that penal concern with drugs began only in the early 1900s. What is less often explicitly recognised is that it was an international project from the outset. Before then states had fought wars in the name of free trade, trade which included the buying and selling of psychoactive drugs, principally opium. During the latter half of the nineteenth century there had been intermittent moral outrage expressed by some British citizens against participation in the opium trade (Bean 1974: 20). However, the lucrative tax revenue, coupled with the realisation that any withdrawal from the market by the British would simply invite increased participation from other players (French, German, American, Russian and Chinese, to name only the most obvious), undermined the persuasiveness of such moral argument. The political economy of free trade set policy rather than any ethical position that could be formulated. The Spanish–American war of 1898, in which the United States vanquished the decaying Spanish empire and thus acquired the Philippines, Guam, Puerto Rico and Cuba, fundamentally altered American geopolitical and economic reality and thus that of the world. The then Secretary of State, John Hay, proclaimed an 'open door' policy for the United States in the lucrative eastern markets where American traders had previously played only a minor part. For the Americans one happy consequence of promoting a curtailment of the opium trade to China was the erosion of European domination of trade in general (Taylor 1969; Nadelmann 1990). Thus, first and foremost, it cannot escape our attention that drug prohibition policies emerged as the United States came to play a role on the global stage. Once the state apparatus of the USA was directly embroiled in controlling territory outside its traditional sphere of influence, global politics were altered in important ways.

Moral entrepreneurship, balance of power politics and the rise of drug prohibition

However, it was not a conspiracy to promote the trading or political interests of the United States abroad that placed drug prohibition on the agenda. Rather, it was a confluence of factors, amongst which were the changed geopolitical relations, but which also, and perhaps more importantly given our concerns here, included the gathering force of the temperance movement in the United States itself. The newly acquired global presence of the USA meant that the indigenous American politics of abstention could be, indeed had to be, acted out on the world stage. It is an historically contingent fact that the United States became a player in world politics more or less at the same time that the temperance movement became a political force in American society. The Prohibition Party was formed in the USA in 1869. Between that time and the enactment of the 18th Amendment to the Constitution in 1919 there was a concerted and growing campaign by temperance reformers to prohibit a range of substances that were widely available (Szasz 1975). Alcohol, marijuana, cocaine, opium and its derivatives had become the targets of moral entrepreneurship within the United States. The period of alcohol prohibition in the USA lasted until 1933 – prohibition of other intoxicants continued to remain entrenched long after. The history of this social and political movement is complex and the way that it intertwined with US statecraft abroad even more so. The person of one Reverend Wilbur Crafts, head of the International Reform Bureau in the United States, clearly embodied the developments with which we are concerned. The IRF was, in Crafts' words, 'a bureau of lectures and literature, for enactment and enforcement of laws against all moral evils, especially the big five: intoxicants, sex abuses, gambling, pugilism, and commercialization of Sunday' (cited in Nadelmann 1990: 506). Using this institutional base, Crafts took it upon himself to shape American policy regarding the opium trade in the Orient. Pressure from the IRF culminated in Senator Henry Cabot Lodge's nurturing of a resolution in the US Senate which forbade the sale of alcohol or opium by American traders to 'aboriginal tribes and uncivilized races' in the Pacific islands in 1901 (Sinclair 1962: 52). Crafts' success is remarkable, given that statesmen of great stature, including Governor William Howard Taft, had *already* conceived a plan to reinstitute the system of regulation for the opium trade previously operated by the Spanish (Nadelmann 1990: 506). Crafts was mainly interested in alcohol prohibition. Not so Dr Hamilton Wright, who, like Crafts, was a non-governmental actor possessed of great energy and determination. Wright's special interest was in drug prohibition and, in order to affect change at home, his mission affected American policy abroad. He was a vociferous campaigner for narcotics criminalisation, astutely managing the presentation of the issue in the mass media of the day and producing something of a moral panic. Adeptly compiling and constructing statistics relating to both the national and international scene, where previously there had been none, his awareness of the broader international theatre was clear early on. In 1910, for example, he wrote a letter to the Episcopal bishop of the Philippines which concerned the theft of opium and cocaine from US military stockpiles there. These stolen supplies were, Wright alleged, destined for resale 'by unscrupulous persons in the medical department' for sale in US cities (Cloyd 1982: 51). Prior to the Shanghai Convention of 1909 Wright collected information on opium use, importation and distribution in the USA and requested that other nations including Persia, Turkey, India, China, France, Germany and Britain attempt to do the same. According to Cloyd (ibid.), in order to mount a successful international conference on drug control Wright had to create an 'emotion display in favour of drug control' and this required that the United States have 'exemplary opium laws as a model for the rest of the world'. The US Congress obliged with legislation in 1909 that prohibited the importation of opium for smoking into the Philippines and the USA. Thus Wright was able to demonstrate that the USA was 'desirous, on the grounds of humanity and for the purpose of promoting social and moral welfare . . . of taking all possible steps for achieving the suppression of the use of opium for smoking with the least possible delay' (quoted in Joint Study Group 1980: 23–4). This legislation was largely symbolic since neither the US nor any other state had the necessary enforcement apparatus. However, armed with this statute from his home country, Wright was in a position to admonish other nations to join the international fight against narcotics. Although this conference did not produce practical legal measures for the control of drugs, it did generate momentum at the international level that could be used for the passage of significant legislation at home. As Cloyd explained it, 'the initially unrelated political conquest of the Pacific became a resource used by the moral entrepreneur in his quest for a national drug law' (1982: 53). That is why Senator James Robert Mann, a spokesman for the bill in the Senate, 'talked about international obligations rather than domestic morality' (Brecher et al. 1972: 49). Wright's ability to create an international display at Shanghai, and later at the International Convention in the Hague in 1912, placed America in the moral vanguard against the narcotics trade and this was highly facilitative of the passage of the Harrison Act of 1914 which was the true harbinger of the American international war on drugs (cf. Renborg 1943: 14).

It is worth pointing out that the United States was a relatively late arrival into the circle of imperial powers and that there was not universal support for foreign adventures amongst Americans, many of whom preferred the doctrine of isolationism and disliked the idea of enhancing the power of the federal state. It is not implausible to suggest that the crusade against international drug trafficking provided the moral cloak necessary to legitimate the move beyond the traditional territorial remit of American manifest destiny, analogous to the moral purpose provided to earlier imperial powers by the activities of Christian missionaries. Indeed, Arnold Taylor has written that 'in its early stages the international campaign [against drugs] might quite appropriately be referred to as a missionary movement – or better still as missionary diplomacy' (1969: 29). However, the development of the politics of temperance was more contingent than the 'missionary position' suggests. The prohibition movement came of age during the progressive era when the US federal government was acquiring some of the character Europeans had long granted to the state. The paternalistic concerns of the prohibitionists struck a responsive cord with significant sectors of the rural 'old stock' America – not generally known for enthusing about the growth of the state apparatus. The separate agendas of the temperance movement and the progressive movement dovetailed, but not by design. During the period of progressivism – and especially during World War I – the US federal government took over many aspects of the economy. It allocated resources, regulated prices, supervised cartels, ran the railroads and commandeered factories. The effort to engineer American society's morality using the power of the federal state came at the zenith of this phase in US history, but the enactment of the 18th Amendment, ushering in prohibition in 1919, was almost exactly co-incident with the end of the progressive era. During the 'Roaring '20s' state planning became subordinated to big business and it was not until Roosevelt's assumption of office in March 1932, which launched the New Deal, that federal planning and control was reinvigorated. The period of ostensible *laissez-faire* governance during the 1920s was one in which the US state attempted to exercise control over the nation's drinking habits and other vices; to little effect, one might add, other than nurturing the syndication of the newly created illicit markets. Piling irony on irony, Roosevelt's administration, which ushered in the era of 'big government', also presided over the repeal of alcohol prohibition. At that point, narcotics prohibition was all that was left as a lasting achievement after sixty years of moral crusades against all manner of vice. The missionary zeal of the drug prohibitionists was nurtured in the entrepreneurial habitus that characterised American industrial capitalism, but this project to police morals was also conditioned by the halting progress of federal state building. The experiment in moral engineering took shape between the contrapuntal developments of the American welfare state and *laissez-faire* capitalism. All the while, American expansionism abroad was developing on a rather different tack from that of previous imperial powers. The United States did not build outward from its all-but-colonies. Hawaii, the Virgin Islands, Puerto Rico, the canal zone at

Panama, and a few scattered military bases like those of Guantánamo were the main territorial acquisitions (the Philippines was made independent in 1946). While the twentieth-century history of United States foreign policy finds the USA brow-beating and arm-twisting other governments, organising coups and fighting wars by proxy, in the main American suzerainty did not equate with territorial annexation. It was largely the power of the purse and the media, of scientists, technicians and corporate executives – not of colonial garrisons or officials – that established American global hegemony. The prohibitionists who rode on the coat-tails of American expansionism were but one contingent in the legion of salesmen who sold American ideas, products and processes around the globe.

The international success of the drug prohibition movement was contingent on other (broadly speaking) transnational factors, not least of which were the perceptions held by many Americans of migratory pressures, perceptions fuelled by fears of racial contagion and miscegenation. In the latter years of the nineteenth century, California was a bloody battleground between immigrants from the Orient and the Occident who competed for employment building the infrastructure on the frontier. The opium laws brought in during that period performed an important symbolic and practical role in this conflict. Control of opium was just one of the many legal devices that were useful in the suppression of Chinese immigrants, and so, Paul Siu (1987) records, 'the victory ultimately fell to the European immigrant and his offspring' (1987: 50). One might add that with this victory came a prohibition against 'oriental' forms of intoxication while alcohol, the preferred intoxicant of Irish and other European pioneers, was less successfully criminalised. Somewhat later, large-scale Mexican immigration across the frontier into the United States facilitated similar control efforts for marijuana (Musto 1973). In the context of this moral panic, Mexicans were depicted as lazy, unreliable, and prone to criminality, attributes that were linked to a perceived propensity to indulge in marijuana smoking. Again, prohibition against this intoxicant facilitated the desire to control a suspect foreign population. Throughout this period Hamilton Wright campaigned on the issue of drug use by 'the negroes' (Cloyd 1982: 53) – images of bullet-proof blacks fuelled the campaign to control illicit drugs in the American south. Thus ethnic divisions and drug prohibition became fused. 'In each case', observes Ethan Nadelmann (1990: 507), 'law enforcement officials, journalists, and political leaders provided sensationalist, albeit largely unsubstantiated, reports of the horrid crimes ostensibly committed under the influence of a particular drug.' The fires of narcotics criminalisation were fanned throughout this period by a per-ceived need to control the (international and internal) migration flows of specific ethnic groups and this provided a crucial element in the argument for prohibition. Michael Lind succinctly summed up the mood of the period, noting that 'mass immigration produced a back-lash by old-Stock Americans' (1995: 78). The fear of being overwhelmed by other ethnic groups struck a harmonious chord with the campaigns of prohibitionists. For a time prohibition of all intoxicants was on the statute books but in the end alcohol, a vice preferred by 'old-stock Americans', was struck off.

We can see how domestic American and international politics con-cerning the control of drugs were intertwined in complex ways. How-ever, not all of the analysis should be confined to the United States. The changing global balance of power was itself an important factor. Nigel South (1997: 936) records that the first penal response to drug use in Britain arose in the context of the war effort during the years 1914–19. Prior to that time a medical discourse had provided *the* lan-guage of control for problem drug use. It was the need to mobilise the population for total war that put penal sanctions on the British menu of control options for the first time. From the latter stages of the nineteenth century there had been a strong moral entrepreneurship in Britain as well, not unlike the American case, but domestically it re-sulted in medical regulation rather than penal measures and inter-nationally its effects were quite weak. Medicalisation remained the pre-eminent control response in the UK until the late 1960s. While it took the conditions of total war to introduce criminal law enforcement onto the menu of control responses in the British context, even then drugs later scheduled for prohibition (notably amphetamines) were used to enhance worker productivity and soldierly effectiveness. In-deed the use of stimulants was an important pharmacological weapon during both wars on all sides (Szasz 1975). All of the industrial pow-ers, including the United States, have made use of the pharmacopoeia to facilitate the waging of war. But that is a mere footnote; the main point to be stressed here is that criminal law enforcement remained a relatively minor option on the menu of control responses in Great Britain until the period of the 1960s.

World War I saw the tide turn against European global hegemony (Toynbee 1939/1962: 43) and this contributed to the gradual global imposition of the American prohibitionist model as well. The contin-gency of fratricidal war in Europe (*la Guerre Totale*), not once but twice within the space of a quarter century, is consequential for the pro-gress of prohibition norms in drug control. Historically the European powers had not been enthusiastic about narcotic control, and what policies were produced focused on medicalisation and regulation rather than prohibition supported by the criminal law. This is clear in the attitude of Germany around the time of the Hague Convention in 1912. This Convention was the first to establish a moral duty to give penal attention to drugs as well as limit their manufacture and distribution. Due to lobbying by Germany, then the leading country in drug manufacturing, the Convention was scripted in such a way that these duties would come into force only after it became effective, which required *universal* signing (Joint Study Group 1980).[3] At that time only the USA, China and (interestingly) the Netherlands were signatories. Indeed, general accession did not happen until after World War I when, at the instigation of the US delegation, the parties signing the Treaty of Versailles simultaneously acceded to the Hague Convention (Renborg 1943: 16). During the inter-war years, the League of Nations provided the framework for much of the discussion, which somewhat limited the role played by the USA, since it was not a participant. However, unilateral efforts by the United States calculated to bring about international drug prohibition continued. In 1931 a convention was passed whereby sanctions against states violating existing treaties on drug-related matters were broadened. This was an extension of the universal applicability requirements already in existence; the evolving drug prohibition regime abutted the international law doctrine of sovereignty bringing it close to becoming a truly transnational control regime. Be that as it may, Harry Anslinger, the US government's vehement spokesperson on drug-related matters, thought the convention too limited. By this time drug prohibition had been thoroughly institutionalised within the state apparatus of the USA. As head of the Federal Bureau of Narcotics, Anslinger played a prominent role in popularising tales of drug-induced crime within the United States, further facilitating the continuing domestic encroachment of federal law enforcement in the United States.[4] Drawing on his experience as head of the foreign control section of the prohibition unit during the late 1920s he played the primary role in pursuing international drug control as well. After World War II, the USA came to dominate the international drug control scene as never before – with the obvious exception of territory beyond the 'iron curtain'. In 1961 New York played host to meetings which codified all the earlier treaties. The United States continued to shepherd the international community of states into a comprehensive international drug prohibition regime. Subsequent landmarks included the 1971 United Nations Convention on Psychotropic Substances and the 1988 United Nations Convention Against Illicit Traffic in Narcotic Drugs and Psychotropic Substances. It should be noted that, while European countries were less able to affect the outcome of these treaty negotiations (having long since been eclipsed by the geopolitical dominance of the USA) some limitations were placed on the prohibition regime. Significantly, the UK, West Germany, Switzerland and the Netherlands (perhaps at the behest of the pharmaceutical companies) secured the insertion into the preamble of the 1971 Convention a statement to the effect that 'the availability for medical and scientific purposes should not be unduly restricted'.[5] Another element of the 1971 Convention, which secured treatment as an *alternative* to punishment, indicates that the punitive prohibitionism did not entirely hold sway (Joint Study Group 1980: 28). This does not mean that Europeans were 'soft on drugs' because, while European governments were not uniformly keen to use the criminal law to control the consumption of illicit drugs, they were more willing to criminalise the trade itself (Pearson 1999).

Contradictions in transnational drug prohibition regimes?

Taylor (1969) provided systematic evidence of the links between narcotic control and US foreign policy in the period up to 1939. After the world wars, when US hegemony (at least in 'the West') was all but indisputable, that tendency continued (Nadelmann 1993: 103). In the second half of the century the new 'internationalist' perspective of the United States required an enhancement of a wide range of its governmental activities abroad, ranging from intelligence, military and economic ventures to diplomatic and foreign aid programmes. It did not escape notice that 'drug control is a label which gives easier access to strategic countries than military espionage or security personnel' (Joint Study Group 1980: 27). In steering the international drug control agenda the USA had created a vehicle for sending policing personnel abroad in numbers never before seen. This fact is perhaps more self-evidently political in Latin America (subject to the Monroe Doctrine) than it is in Europe (the recipient of Marshall Aid). Although the figures are not easy to interpret, it appears that, from the 1960s onwards, the number of authorised US overseas 'law enforcement' personnel greatly surpassed the number of conventional overseas 'secret service' posts (Nadelmann 1993: 479–81, 482, 486). Thus, 'seen in the context of overall foreign policy, it is not very surprising that France has been the initiator of European regional activity, for France is *always* countervailing US power in Europe in order to stress its own central position in an independent Europe' (Joint Study Group 1980:

28). It seems fair to suggest that the European embrace of drug criminalisation and penal prohibition was brought about by policy considerations other than those aimed at mediating, modifying and managing drug use. Seen as a domestic issue, drugs appear as a 'low policing' function or a public health issue. In the context of international relations, policing drug prohibition became an issue of 'high policing'. It is probably incorrect to assume, as some criminologists have been wont to, that the establishment of the Pompidou Group in 1971 was a signal that European policy-makers had come around to the prohibitionist's view that criminalisation was the *sine qua non* of effective drug policy. It was not simply a case of 'if you can't beat them, join them'. Rather, taking cognisance of the 'high policing' issues involved, the more apt aphorism might be: 'fight fire with fire'.

Examining the different tenor of drug prohibition in Europe and in the Americas, the United States' traditional sphere of influence, is productive of insights into the contemporary transnational state system. For example, some have detected stark contradictions in US policies in Latin America. Peter Andreas (1995) observed that promotion of the neo-liberal agenda by the US required a curtailment of state intervention, while promotion of drug prohibition required an escalation of state intervention and, according to him, this set of policies was working at cross-purposes. He put his view to a US House of Representatives Subcommittee on Crime in 1996:

> The unleashing of market forces has unintentionally encouraged and facilitated not only legal economic activity, but illegal economic activity as well. Part of the problem is that legal and illegal markets are increasingly intertwined . . . The logic of liberal economic theory, after all, is for the State to conform to the dictates of the market. Although illegal, the drug economy should be seen as part of this process. Neoclassical economics suggests that countries should specialise in exports in which they enjoy a comparative advantage. For some countries this has meant their market niche in exporting illegal drugs.
>
> (US Committee on the Judiciary 1996: 59–60)

Andreas argued that these contradictions were maintained through 'institutionalised denial' that was facilitated by an institutional separation of drug control and economic policy considerations. However, US foreign policy in the Americas may not be as contradictory as it appears. Looking at United Nations reports on international drug trafficking one cannot help but see an instance of what sociologists of development used to call the 'north–south divide'. One such report (UNDCP 1994) evinces a near exclusive concern with control of the export market from the Andean region, South-west and South-east Asia to North America and Europe. This pattern of north–south relations is cartographically depicted in a report of the United Nations Drug Control Programme (UNDCP 1997). The series of maps provided in this report clearly illustrate that it is high value (illicit) commodities from the southern 'developing countries' that are the principal target of drug prohibition. This pattern of control response is evident in precursor chemical seizures, an 'indirect indicator' of the size of the illicit market in psychoactive substances. The UNDCP report (1994) notes, tellingly, that 'most of the precursors seized are used for cocaine production, followed to a lesser extent, by precursors needed for heroin production. In contrast, there were few reported seizures, by frequency and amount, of the precursors for LSD and MDA/MDMA precursors than might be expected from the apparently increasing availability of the respective drugs' (p. 11). The sheer concentration of effort to control this export trade from the under-developed south to the developed north can be readily interpreted in terms of an attempt to preserve capitalist relations between 'core and periphery', or 'metropolis and hinterland', that have characterised north–south relations since decolonisation began. This, of course, raises questions about the extent to which prohibition against commodities such as heroin and cocaine has been partly motivated by 'monetary nationalism' stemming from 'balance of payments' concerns (see Roxborough 1979 for a general discussion of concepts relating to underdevelopment). Seen in the context of north–south relations the announcement by US President Clinton of a $1.3 billion aid package in order to help Colombia's military establish two new 'anti-narcotics battalions' appears as a resounding twenty-first-century reaffirmation of the Monroe Doctrine. Despite strong arguments for alternative strategies (Nadelmann 1988), significant vested interests embedded in the transnational political-economic system entail criminal law prohibition backed up by military force.

Tensions in drug control policy within the context of the European Union are rather different. In that regional context a distinction between two levels of drug control has been operant. At the 'low end' – control of drug users and user/dealers – there has historically been a variety of control responses. As evidence of this Nick Dorn (1998: 11) pointed to the 'acidic' debates between France and the Netherlands, those between Denmark and 'her more temperance-minded Nordic *sister nations*' and the differing levels of enforcement against cannabis users in the various Länder of Germany. In his, and others', estimations this variety is an entrenched feature of European drug policy which emanates from the distinctive cultural differences across the territory of the EU (Dorn et al. 1996). However, at the 'high end', where the European Union 'faces outward', there is a marked convergence of efforts, techniques and aims. In the 1990s, convergence of policy and practice in enforcement against drug importation and trafficking was reinforced by an increasing use of criminal law sanctions, themselves of increasing intensity, supplemented by administrative or civil law measures, that is: asset confiscation (Dorn 1998: 7–8). By the late 1990s it was clear to knowledgeable observers that action against drug trafficking had become *the* site for the convergence of policing systems in Europe as anti-terrorist police co-operation had been in the 1970s (Anderson 1993). In other words, the system of drug law enforcement had become integral to the European security apparatus. The perceived contradictions between high and low policing of drug markets in Europe were the product of the political need to establish a governable territory with a unified global face. Attempting to introduce 'harm reduction' type approaches at the low end in the context of high-level drug prohibition is not without its difficulties, of course. Drug law enforcement definitions of 'victory' (for example those associated with crackdowns, interdiction and other 'supply-side' tactics) may eclipse definitions of success associated with public health and 'harm reduction'. This tension has been well documented in Australia (Maher and Dixon 1999). Nevertheless, as Nigel South pointed out, an ana-lysis of European drug policy 'demonstrates how much more there is to the formulation of drug policy than a US-inspired "war"' (1999: 655), perhaps suggesting that prohibition could be somehow modified. Others seemed to think so (Albrecht and van Kalmthout 1989). However, while academic criminologists in Europe called for depenalisation of drugs, Jürgen Storbeck, Director General of Europol, called for a shift of resources away from local (i.e. low) policing in order to tackle the security threat posed to Europe by a rising tide of organised crime, a significant proportion of which he associated with drug markets (Storbeck 1999). The intergovernmental responsibilities assumed by the EU in the 1990s have constituted Europe as a 'security community' of which the apparatus of drug enforcement is an integral feature (Anderson et al. 1995: 161–4).

During the 1990s there arose a clear recognition among most policy analysts in the drugs field that 'drug policy is never purely about drugs' (Dorn 1998: 11). From about that time the literature dedicated to analysing the transnational dimensions of drug law enforcement began to develop in earnest. Ethan Nadelmann's, cited throughout this chapter, is an obvious example of this. It seems worth pointing out that, as a scholar, Nadelmann did not fly the flag of criminology, but rather gained a foothold in the academy in the field of politics and international relations. Working in an economic vein, Peter Reuter examined the effects of drug enforcement on criminal markets, demonstrating that their 'disorganised' nature was due to the effects of law enforcement itself (Reuter 1983). This did much to clarify the effects of law enforcement tactics on the American drug market, showing how many of their negative attributes (for example, the associated violence) are the result of the tactical deployment of law enforcement in the service of prohibition rather than an attribute of drug use itself. Further, Reuter's work with others also demonstrated that even a major increase in drug interdiction at the US border would not significantly reduce drug consumption in the United States (Reuter et al. 1988) – a fact which did little to affect policy. In 1996 the USA embarked on a significant programme for 'stiffening borders' which was announced by President Bill Clinton in a State of the Union Address (Sheptycki 1998: 493). Reuter continued to press his analysis into the domain of foreign policy (1992) but his vision was lacking strategic outlook. This was not the case with the work of Tom Naylor (1996). Also working from within an economics perspective he produced an insightful analysis which, like Andreas (1995), was quite corrosive of the assumed demarcations between the licit and illicit economy. Transposing these insights to the transnational realm led Naylor to document the involvement of a variety of law enforcement and intelligence services around the world in an array of criminal offences including predatory crimes, money laundering and smuggling which nicely dovetailed with some of the observations of the political scientists (Naylor 1999). The conclusion? The political economy of drug prohibition is a strange brew indeed. As high policing and military institutions come to involve themselves with the practices of global drug prohibition the more secretive and élitist ethos of the security services gains ground and the ideal of a transparent, rule-governed and politically neutral transnational system becomes less viable (Bigo 1994; Anderson et al. 1995; Sheptycki 1997: 133). The drug prohibition regime becomes correspondingly difficult to change. Drug policy is indeed about more than drugs, but in order to grasp this requires that we think outside the usual disciplinary boundaries.

The transnational system and drug prohibition

By the latter years of the twentieth century drug prohibition had become the paradigm example of a transnational regime based on global criminal law creation. Transnational because, although drug prohibition was the product of campaigning from within the United States, campaigning which reached its apotheosis in the moment when American global hegemony appeared to reach its height, it had become a regime integral to the fabric of a transnational system *qua* system. It seems important to emphasise at this point that, in the post-Cold War era, that system came to be based in a more multi-polar balance of state power than previously. The transnational system developed its own bureaucracy existing 'above' that of the apparatuses of nation-states. This bureaucracy should be understood as both directive of, and directed by, the state-system that underpins it. It represents a 'pooling of sovereignty' since transnational institutions 'supersede the power of their constituent states, in varying degrees, constituting a *de facto* global bureaucracy' (Castells 1997: 269). Insofar as a specific transnational regime is empowered by notions of 'universal applicability' (which, to a significant extent, drug prohibition is) it can be more directive than directed in relations with states parties. In the 1990s the United Nations stressed 'the importance of national and international action to implement the provisions of the international drug control treaties' (INCB 1994: 2) and the International Narcotics Control Board argued that:

> The functioning of the international drug control system depends on the universal application of the provisions of the international drug control treaties. Deficiencies in national legislation and/or in the implementation of national laws and regulations create loopholes in the global network of protective measures. The board invites Governments to up-date their national legislation in line with the international drug control treaties and to ensure that implementation of that legislation and encourages them to request assistance from the United Nations International Drug Control programme for those purposes.
>
> (p. 2)

This is not to underestimate the continuing importance of states, the USA in particular. Richard Haas (1999) has argued that building and maintaining a stable international order 'requires sustained effort by the world's most powerful actor, the United States' (p. 41). American predominance is not uncontested, but we are not considering the *general* characteristics of the transnational system and the relative importance of state's interests within it. Rather our attention focuses on but one aspect, having to do with drug prohibition. In this realm the legacy of moral entrepreneurship that characterised American actions at home and abroad at the beginning of the century remained operant at its end. As the century drew to a close one state, at least, remained pivotal in the maintenance of what, otherwise, had become a truly transnational control regime. US domestic policy towards drug use was scripted long ago by a 'prohibitive' philosophy (Zimring and Hawkins 1997), a logic that was subsequently entrenched in the transnational drug control regime.

Drug prohibition was initially the product of actions by non-state actors and was later promoted by sub-state agents. Both types of actors, in various ways, have shaped transnational drug control subsequently. It is much regretted that we do not better understand the role played by pharmaceutical companies in the shaping of the transnational regulation of drugs. The limitations of the empirical record aside, the conceptual point is that the actions of non-state and sub-state agents are often misunderstood or underplayed within the 'billiard-ball model' of international relations theory. The term 'transnational' itself stands as a necessary corrective to this (see the Introduction to this volume). This is important in the contemporary period when non-state personnel and institutions are again shaping the world-wide control regime relating to drugs. In the 1980s, at the apparent height of American global suzerainty, European academics were pessimistic about the prospects for reform of drug prohibition away from a punitive model. The view taken was that, partly because of bureaucratic intransigence and partly because of the 'moral commitment' of many persons who occupy positions of importance in the transnational control regime, it was very difficult to shift the focus away from punitive prohibition towards a model of tolerance and harm reduction (Joint Study Group 1980: 33–7, 257–61). However intransigent the global bureaucracy might be, the abiding irony which continued to dog its efforts to prohibit the drug trade and drug use is that, despite well-publicised successes against limited targets, there has not been a successful eradication of any mass-market drug (Mitchell 1991: 181; O'Malley and Mugford 1994).[6] Thus have emerged oppositional forces to criminalisation from non-governmental agents and even some states. An example of the former is the Lindesmith Centre, a product of the Open Society Foundation established by George Soros a man who made his fortune in currency speculation. Soros might be likened to the morale entrepreneurs who first embarked on drug prohibition, but this moralism is that of neo-liberal cosmopolitanism. In this view, drug prohibition is an ideological chimera and the moral battle to be waged is against the harm that the drug war itself causes (Soros 1997; Baker 1999). It is too soon to say if a new breed of moral entrepreneur might tip the balance away from the punitive model towards one of toleration and harm reduction. One indicator that it might is the suggestion that the more multi-polar the balance of state-power becomes in the global system, the less assured becomes the preferred model of one state, even the *seigneur*. Against this it might be argued that, after one hundred years of reiteration about the need for prohibition, the criminalisation rationale that has driven the drug control regime for so long is now unassailable. After all, despite its contradictions, most of the big global state powers subscribe to the criminalisation model. This is difficult to weigh up. Switzerland has experimented successfully with heroin prescription as a means of minimising the social harm connected with that type of drug use. Dutch 'tolerance', pragmatic and contradictory as it is (Mol and Trautmann 1991), has spread to many German cities and is a *de facto* policy in other regions across northern Europe. The antipodes have also started to experiment with responses that de-emphasise the part that criminal law needs to play (O'Malley 1999). These developments have produced a bevy of new agents acting transnationally, raising derision among the ranks of the 'traditional' prohibitionists. For example, an article in the *Journal of Substance Abuse Treatment* (Satel and Aeschbach 1999) portrayed the scientists who carried out the Swiss heroin experiment as 'travelling abroad to promote [rather than present] their findings'. This article suggested, further, that the Swiss Federal Office of Public Health was not motivated to sponsor scientific enquiry as a responsible reaction by public health officials and clinical practitioners to a social problem. Rather, it was suggested, in terms not far off hyperbole, that the Swiss Parliament, expressly linked to the 'harm reduction and legalization movements' (sic), was attempting blanket decriminalisation of drug consumption. At the end of the twentieth century the balance of forces was thus set. The dynamic tensions inherent in the many contradictions of the drug control regime were acute enough that historical contingency, fumbling chance and accident might play a future role in the reformation of the transnational drug control regime.

Having said that, non-state actors, and actors whose normal function is at the domestic level, all operate transnationally within the context of balance of state-power politics. At this level the drug control regime is understood to contribute to the stability of the transnational state system. Thus, the opening paragraph of the 1993 Report of the International Narcotics Control Board reported that 'during the last two decades, the world has witnessed the "globalisation" of the drug abuse problem and the situation has worsened drastically' (INCB 1994: 1). Further, 'Governments are beginning to realise that international cooperation in drug control, which in the past was an expression of solidarity, has now become a matter of urgent self-defence' (ibid.). Foreign policy analysts have noted how co-operation in the international war on drugs attained a new importance in state-security discourses in the post-Cold War period as 'narco-diplomacy' replaced anti-communism as the guiding rationale for security agencies around the world (Griffith 1994). The drug war has seemingly become inextricable from the concerns of state security and therefore a matter of 'high policing'. In such circumstances it is not easy to see that public health officials possess the requisite expertise to substantially change the character of the transnational control regime.

Transnationalisation, policing and drugs: a summary

It is impossible to do justice to the complexities of this transnational political history in a short overview such as this and, indeed, the social consequences of prohibition have not been examined at all. This overview has had the more limited aim of displaying some of the salient facets and contingencies that underscored the development of the transnational drug prohibition regime. This was undertaken to illustrate the utility of the transnational perspective in understanding the development of one element of contemporary policing: the 'drug war'. It is thought that a more general understanding of transnational policing issues might emerge from looking at the prototypical instance of transnational law enforcement. Therefore, three points emerging from this overview are worth stressing. One thing amply demonstrated is the importance of non-state actors in the evolution of international drug prohibition and, by implication, within transnational policing generally. In the early years of this century no state representative seriously thought to embark on such a project. It was the concerted efforts of moral entrepreneurs outside the normal state apparatus who put the drug issue on the agenda. Non-state actors help shape the transnational system in important ways that realist theories of international relations seldom try to account for. Our understanding of the part played by such agents needs to be sharpened, not only in relation to drug prohibition, but across the whole range of policing activities. It is hoped that research on these questions will be stimulated in order that the future shaping of the transnational police enterprise, and the transnational state system more generally, might be better understood.

In the contemporary period new non-state actors have entered the debate and it will be important to study them as the forms of transnational governance continue to develop and be elaborated. This overview also demonstrates the role of sub-state actors in the continuing evolution of international drug prohibition. Harry Anslinger, the first head of the Federal Bureau of Narcotics, was in charge of a domestic agency and his efforts in the 1930s to shape international responses to drug use were not being pursued through entirely normal diplomatic channels. He was not, in his capacity as head of the FBN, a sovereign representative of his country abroad, hence the designation 'sub-state actor'. While it is true to say that Anslinger's goals were in accord with the general drift of official American foreign policy at the time he was nevertheless, in his capacity as director of an agency with domestic competence, a sub-state actor playing a role in international affairs. This distinction may be easily overlooked in this specific instance, but the potential for sub-state agents to create diplomatic problems should not be, as the case of Operation Casablanca detailed in chapter five of this volume well illustrates. Systematic attention to the sometimes complementary and sometimes contrary actions of sub-state and sovereign-state-actors as they play their roles on the global stage is necessary for a comprehensive understanding of the transnational system. High-level officials, that is those officials who do represent the sovereign power of their states in international affairs, pay scant attention to the international activities of these types of agents except, of course, when those activities attain some political significance, attract media attention or disrupt foreign relations (Nadelmann 1993: 108). Since these sub-agents are the principal motors of the transnational drug control regime, and transnational policing more generally, clearly it would not do for academics to mirror the myopia of those senior officials.

Lastly, the gradual assimilation of drug prohibition as integral to the interests of state security and the security of the transnational state system raises general questions about the role played by agencies traditionally associated with the 'high police' function that have not been sufficiently answered. Academic inquiry about policing will have to move beyond the narrow focus on national and municipal police actions, and the preoccupation with uniformed patrol and detective work, if it is to accurately assess the relative importance of 'high' and 'low' policing functions. This historical synopsis indicates the fusion of balance of power politics and foreign policy realism in the evolution of transnational drug control. The tensions that exist between policies directed at public health and security policy need to be brought out into the light of day if we are to understand the past and affect the future of the drug control regime. It hardly needs to be said that other aspects of the transnational policing architecture will be differentially affected by the interests of state security; transnational governance, it seems, does not obviate 'high' policing, it elevates it.

Some general lessons

Some analysts of the contemporary global scene have noted the alignment of business and political interests in the reconstruction of nation-based state power at a 'higher level'. The transnational level is the only level where a degree of control of global flows of wealth, information and power can be exercised (Streeck and Schmitter 1991; Thurow 1993; Castells 1997). Aspects of this institutional framework of the transnational system are quite well developed and readers will no doubt be familiar with many of the acronyms that festoon the transnational bureaucracy (WTO, IMF, OECD, G7, etc.). It is important to look at how these transnational bureaucracies are themselves governed because they appear to be effectively insulated from the people whose interests they purport to represent (Castells 1997: 309–49). This volume has looked at issues that arise from one specific sector of global governance, the transnational police enterprise. Questions about how transnational policing is held to account politically are no less important than questions about the governance of the global system generally for it appears that, in this realm too, there is something of a democratic deficit (Sheptycki 1996).

What the history of drug prohibition outlined above shows is that the development of a transnational control regime is subject to contingency and depends in important ways on the actions of non-state actors. The result is that it is not easy to make predictions about future developments in transnational governance. This overview also shows that, once created, a transnational enterprise of any scope is difficult to repeal or reform. Accordingly, transnational policing will likely continue to focus on drug prohibition for the foreseeable future. Furthermore, as Frank Gregory's contribution to this volume amply illustrates, international agenda-setting in the criminal justice sphere is slow and uneven. Campaigners in ecological non-governmental organisations must view this as a challenge. There are also victims of state aggression who might benefit from more vigorous policing of human rights abuses, and so human rights organisations must *continue* to think about policing issues (Sheptycki 2000). It has been pointed out elsewhere that a variety of 'folk devils' provide the rationale for fostering a transnational police enterprise (Sheptycki 1995). Despoilers of the environment and traders in endangered species jostle for headlines with child-sex tourists and fissile materials smugglers. There are others who already have priority in the transnational policing effort: terrorists, fraudsters, drugs, weapons and human smugglers. A moral case can be made for policing in each of these instances. However, it is not a simple matter to weigh priorities and, given the complexity of the decision-making processes of the transnational system, the rationale calculus of prioritisation will inevitably be fraught. States' interests, especially the interests of states who would be global suzerains, remain an important factor, and this raises persistent questions about the exact role played by agencies of 'high policing' in the evolution of the transnational state system. All of these calculations are made more difficult by the fact that transnational governance is not reducible to the state-centred or state-security preoccupations of old-fashioned international relations discourses. As Les Johnston's contribution to this book makes evident, private policing is also being undertaken globally. The actions of non-state institutions are likely to shape certain important features of the transnational policing enterprise as well and these require scholarly attention. All the while these issues are being refracted through the eye of global media, which are not wholly beholden to any particular interests save, for the most part, their own commercial ones. The endless kaleidoscope of 'infotainment' purveyed by the mass media has created a sense of powerlessness. Moreover, Manning's broad survey of issues rising out of the 'information society' shows that there are manifold contradictions that arise when considering transnational policing. The intersection of computer technology, the internet and other interactive technologies of data manipulation, surveillance and communication, as well as the business of intellectual property, produces no clear evidence of the liberating potential of the new technologies – on the contrary what we discover are the strange contradictions of policing in the information society. Castells has cited one survey showing that there is 'no clear direction in the public's political thinking other than frustration with the current system and an eager responsiveness to alternative political solutions and appeals' (Castells 1997: 343). The political alienation, of which this is a symptom, may give moral entrepreneurs new opportunities to exploit possibilities and build and/or reshape global institutions of control. Moral entrepreneurs may, for example, seek to foster a control regime to protect the high seas from those who would profit from the dumping of toxic waste, a development that many would applaud. Other moral entrepreneurs might fixate on issues of less universal benefit. Successful transnational control regimes require universal applicability and so the outcome of these processes is of great interest to all.

It is too soon to tell what sort of global society the contemporary processes of transnationalisation foreshadow. In seeking to do so, an examination of policing on the global stage is of more than particular interest. As the nation-state system gives way to the transnational state system, policing (still largely embedded in nation-states) becomes a barometer of the transnationalisation of governance. As Jean-Paul Brodeur showed in chapter two, parochial politics form the backdrop to contemporary dramas of transnational policing, but that should not deflect attention from the transnational stage itself. The future evolution of transnational policing practice will be facilitated by a combination of bureaucratic decision-making of Byzantine complexity fuelled by the energies of entrepreneurs (guided by the idiosyncracies of their own moral compasses) who fixate on a wide variety of issues. It will also be the partial product of the transnational networks of police agents that are already in place, as Didier Bigo makes clear in chapter three. The array of interests that circumscribe the transnational state system are not easy to fathom. To do so requires a window onto that system, and social researchers who take policing (transnational and otherwise) as their subject of study can expect a good view. Provided, that is, that policing is broadly defined. Understood as a set of practices that underscore, weave into and patrol the very basis of governance itself there seems little doubt that issues in transnational policing will continue to occupy the attention of theorists, policy-makers, and moral entrepreneurs in the decades to come.

Notes

1 The synoptic history of drug prohibition that follows owes its inspiration to this document. This chapter is dedicated to the memory of Derick McClintock, one of the chief architects of the project which this document reports. The author would like to thank Karim Murji who read and commented on an earlier draft of this chapter.

2 The view that drug control was the prototype for international control regimes was understood relatively early on. For example, Bertil Renborg (1943) noted that the 'study of the international drug control shows that as a result of international co-operation and legislation a whole industry in its national and international aspects has been strictly regulated. National interests have been superseded by international interests. States have submitted to far-reaching international regulations.' He went on to suggest that, *mutatis mutandis*, it 'appears logical to suggest that drug control might serve as a model and example for other fields of activity which may require international control' (p. 277).

3 Renborg (1943: 3–4) hints darkly about the inhibitory pressure against the campaign for international prohibition from the 'financial interests represented by manufacturing industries and trading concerns', but does not elaborate on their national specificities. There was, and continues to be, resistance to the anti-narcotic legislative drive from within the American medical and pharmacology establishment which was argued on the grounds of efficacy. Articles in leading American medical journals in the first half of the twentieth century made plain that 'instead of improving conditions the laws recently passed have made the problem more complex' (Brecher et al. 1972: 50). It appears that, where resistance by medical practitioners or the pharmaceutical industry to criminalisation is at all successful, it is depicted by drug prohibitionists as animated by the profit motive.

4 Indeed, Anslinger took credit for circulating many stories about the connection between crime and cannabis that would seem out of all proportion to many people today. He wrote that 'much of the irrational juvenile violence and killing that has written a new chapter of shame and tragedy is traceable directly to this hemp intoxication'. Thus 'I knew action had to be taken to get proper control legislation passed'. So by 1937, 'under my direction, the bureau launched two important steps: first, a legislative plan to seek from Congress a new law that would place Marihuana and its distribution directly under federal control. Secondly, on radio and at major forums, such as that presented annually by the *New York Herald Tribune*, I told the story of this evil weed of the fields and riverbeds and roadsides. I wrote articles for magazines; our agents gave hundreds of lectures to parents, educators, social and civic leaders. In network broadcasts I reported on the growing list of crime, including murder and rape. I described the nature of Marihuana and its close kinship to hashish. I continued to hammer at the facts. I believe we did a thorough job, for the public was alerted and the laws to protect them were passed both nationally and at the state level' (quoted in Schofield 1971: 45–6). As Michael Schofield further remarked, 'Anslinger's influence as a hyperactive reformer went far beyond the boundaries of the United States. He was the American representative at many international meetings and at others he was able to exert considerable pressure on the delegates as the Commissioner of the Treasury Department's Bureau of Narcotics. It was also well known that the main financial support for these international organizations came from the United States' (p. 46). Alfred Lindesmith later felt moved to object to the manipulation of the evidence by the Narcotics Bureau under Anslinger's direction. Nevertheless, the inclusion of cannabis into international agreements mainly concerned with opiates and cocaine 'was largely due to the efforts of one determined man, combined with inadequate research methods in the countries where the drugs were most prevalent and the ignor-ance of other delegates from countries where cannabis at that time was largely unknown' (p. 47).

5 I am grateful to Peggy Dwyer for drawing my attention to the 'horse trading' attempted by various pharmaceutical interests that went on behind the scenes at this conference. The results of her research are awaited with great anticipation.

6 Some see this as the Achilles heel of drug prohibition logic. As Gregory pointed out in chapter four, there should be five evolutionary stages in the

development of any prohibition regime: (1) activity lawful, (2) activity redefined as a problem, (3) agitation for suppression and criminalisation, (4) activity becomes criminal offence and (5) hopefully, activity significantly decreases. The hundred-year war against drugs has not yet reached phase five. Indeed conditions have worsened and some are wont to argue that this is so precisely because of the attempt at prohibition.

References

Albrecht, H.-J. and van Kalmthout, A. (1989) 'European Perspectives on Drug Policies', in H.-J. Albrecht and A. van Kalmthout (eds), *Drug Policies in Western Europe*, Freiburg im Breisgau: Max-Planck-Institut für Ausländisches und Internationales Strafrecht.

Anderson, M. (1993) 'The United Kingdom and Organised Crime – the International Dimension', *European Journal of Crime, Criminal Law and Criminal Justice*, Vol. 1, No. 4, pp. 292–308.

Anderson, M., den Boer, M., Cullen, P., Gilmore, W., Raab, C., and Walker, N. (1995) *Policing the European Union: Theory, Law and Practice*, Oxford: Clarendon Press.

Andreas, P. (1995) 'Free-market Reform and Drug Market Prohibition: US Policies at Cross-purposes in Latin America', *Third World Quarterly*, Vol. 16, No. 1, pp. 75–87.

Baker, R. (1999) 'A Philanthropist Defies Drug War Orthodoxy', *The Nation*, 20 September.

Bean, P. (1974) *The Social Control of Drugs*, London: Martin Robertson.

Bertram, E., Blackman, K., Sharpe, K. and Andreas, P. (1996) *Drug War Politics*, Berkeley: University of California Press.

Bigo, D. (1994) 'The European Internal Security Field: Stakes and Rivalries in a Newly Developing Area of Police Intervention', in M. Anderson and M. den Boer (eds), *Policing Across National Boundaries*, London: Pinter.

Brecher, E. M. and the Editors of Consumer Reports (1972) *Licit and Illicit Drugs: The Consumers Union Report on Narcotics, Stimulants, Inhalants, Hallucinogens and Marijuana – including Caffeine, Nicotine and Alcohol*, Boston: Little, Brown and Co.

Castells, M. (1997) *The Power of Identity*, Oxford: Basil Blackwell.

Cloyd, J. W. (1982) *Drugs and Information Control: The Role of Men and Manipulation in the Control of Drug Trafficking*, Westport CN: Greenwood Press.

Dorn, N. (1998) 'Editorial: Drug Policies and the European Union', *Drugs: Education, Prevention and Policy*, Vol. 5, No. 1, pp. 5–13.

Dorn, N., Jepsen, J. and Savona, E. (1996) *Drug Policies and Enforcement*, London: Macmillan.

The Economist (1999) 'Citizens Groups: The Non-governmental Order', 11–17 December, pp. 22–4.

Grazia, J. (1991) *DEA: The War against Drugs*, London: BBC Books.

226   *James Sheptycki*

Griffith, I. L. (1994) 'From Cold War Geopolitics to Post-Cold War Geonarcotics', *International Journal of the Canadian Institute of International Affairs*, Special Issue, *Narco-Diplomacy*, Vol. 49, No. 1, pp. 1–36.
Haas, R. (1999) 'What to Do with American Primacy', *Foreign Affairs*, September–October, pp. 37–49.
INCB (1994) *Report of the International Narcotics Control Board for 1993*, Vienna: United Nations, 28 March.
Joint Study Group (1980) *Working Papers of the Joint Study Group on Alcohol and Drugs Control Policy in Great Britain, West Germany and the Netherlands*, Professors L. Hulsman, D. McClintock and S. Quensel presiding, Rotterdam: Universiteitsbibliotheek.
Lind, M. (1995) *The Next American Nation*, New York: The Free Press.
Maher, L. and Dixon, D. (1999) 'Policing and Public Health: Law Enforcement and Harm Minimization in a Street-level Drug Market', *British Journal of Criminology*, Vol. 39, No. 4, pp. 488–512.
Mitchell, C. N. (1991) 'Narcotics: A Case Study in Criminal Law Creation', in J. Gladstone, R. Ericson and C. Shearing (eds), *Criminology, A Readers Guide*, Toronto: Centre of Criminology, University of Toronto.
Mol, R. and Trautmann, K. (1991) 'The Liberal Image of the Dutch Drug Policy', *International Journal on Drug Policy*, Vol. 2, No. 5, pp. 16–21.
Musto, D. (1973) *The American Disease: Origins of Narcotic Control*, New Haven CT: Yale University Press.
Nadelmann, E. (1988) 'US Drug Policy: A Bad Export', *Foreign Policy*, No. 70, Spring, pp. 83–108.
Nadelman, E. (1990) 'Global Prohibition Regimes: The Evolution of Norms in International Society' *International Organization*, Vol. 44, No. 4, pp. 479–526.
Nadelmann, E. (1993) *Cops Across Borders: the Internationalization of US Criminal Law Enforcement*, University Park PA: Pennsylvania State University Press.
Naylor, R. T. (1996) 'From Underworld to Underground: Enterprise Crime, Informal Sector Business and Public Policy Response', *Crime, Law and Social Change*, Vol. 24.
Naylor, R. T. (1999) *Patriots and Profiteers: On Economic Warfare, Embargo-Busting and State-Sponsored Crime*, Toronto: University of Toronto Press.
O'Malley, P. (1999) 'Consuming Risks: Harm Minimization and the Government of Drug Users', in R. Smandych (ed.), *Governable Places: Readings on Governmentality*, Aldershot: Dartmouth.
O'Malley, P. and Mugford, S. (1994) 'The Demand for Intoxicating Commodities: Implications for the "War on Drugs"', *Social Justice*, Vol. 18, No. 4, pp. 49–75.
Pearson, G. (1999) 'Drugs at the End of the Century: Editorial Introduction', *British Journal of Criminology*, Special Issue *Drugs at the End of the Century*, Vol. 39, No. 4, pp. 477–87.

Renborg, B. A. (1943) *International Drug Control: A Study of International Administration by and through the League of Nations*, Washington DC: Carnegie Endowment for International Peace.

Reuter, P. (1983) 'Disorganised Crime: The Economics of the Visible Hand', Cambridge MA: MIT Press.

Reuter, P. (1992) 'The Limits and Consequences of US Foreign Drug Control Efforts', *The Annals of the American Academy*, Vol. 521, pp. 151–62.

Reuter, P., Crawford, G., Cave, J., Murphy, P., Henry, D., Lisowski, W. and Wainstein, E. (1988) *Sealing the Borders: The Effects of Increased Military Participation in Drug Interdiction*, Santa Monica CA: RAND Institute Report.

Roxborough, I. (1979) *Theories of Underdevelopment*, London: Macmillan.

Satel, S. and Aesbach, E. (1999) 'The Swiss Heroin Trial, Scientifically Sound?', *Journal of Substance Abuse Treatment*, Vol. 17, No. 4, pp. 331–5.

Schofield, M. (1971) *The Strange Case of Pot*, Harmondsworth: Penguin.

Sheptycki, J. W. E. (1995) 'Transnational Policing and the Makings of a Postmodern State', *British Journal of Criminology*, Vol. 35, No. 4, pp. 613–35.

Sheptycki, J. W. E. (1996) 'Law Enforcement, Justice and Democracy in the Transnational Arena: Reflections on the War on Drugs', *International Journal of the Sociology of Law*, Vol. 24, No. 1, pp. 61–75.

Sheptycki, J. W. E. (1997) 'Transnationalism, Crime Control and the European State System', *International Criminal Justice Review*, Vol. 7, pp. 130–40.

Sheptycki, J. W. E. (1998) 'Policing, Postmodernism and Transnationalism', *British Journal of Criminology*, Vol. 38, No. 3, pp. 485–503.

Sheptycki, J. W. E. (ed.) (2000) *Policing and Human Rights: A Policing and Society Special Issue*, with contributions from the Vera Institute of Justice, Vol. 10, No. 1.

Sinclair, A. (1962) *Prohibition: The Era of Excess*, London: Faber and Faber.

Siu, P. (1987) *The Chinese Laundryman: A Study of Social Isolation*, New York: New York University Press.

Soros, G. (1997) 'The Drug War Debate: The Drug War "Cannot Be Won": It's Time to Just Say No to Self-destructive Prohibition', *Washington Post*, Sunday, 2 February, Outlook, P1–C1.

South, N. (1997) 'Drugs: Use, Crime and Control', in M. Maguire, R. Morgan and R. Reiner (eds), *The Oxford Handbook of Criminology*, Oxford: Clarendon Press.

South, N. (1999) 'Review Article on European Drug Policy', *British Journal of Criminology*, Vol. 39, No. 4, pp. 654–5.

Storbeck, J. (1999) *Organised Crime in the European Union – The Role of Europol in International Law-Enforcement Co-operation*, The 1999 Police Foundation Lecture, London: Police Foundation.

Streeck, W. and Schmitter, P. (1991) 'From National Corporatism to Trans-national Pluralism: Organised Interests in the Single European Market', *Politics and Society*, Vol. 19, No. 2, pp. 133–64.

228   *James Sheptycki*

Szasz, T. (1975) *Ceremonial Chemistry: The Ritual Persecution of Drugs, Addicts and Pushers,* London: Routledge and Kegan Paul.

Taylor, A. H. (1969) *American Diplomacy and the Narcotics Traffic 1900– 1939: A Study in International Humanitarian Reform,* Durham NC: Duke University Press.

Thurow, L. (1993) *Head to Head: The Coming Economic Battle among Japan, Europe and America,* London: Nicholas Brealey.

Toynbee, A. (1939/1962) *A Study of History,* Vol. 5, *The Disintegration of Civilizations, Part 1,* London: Oxford University Press.

United Nations Drug Control Programme (UNDCP) (1994) *Present Status of Knowledge on the Illicit Drug Industry,* ACC Sub-Committee on Drug Control, Vienna, September 1994 (unpublished document).

United Nations Drug Control Programme (UNDCP) (1997) *World Drug Report,* Oxford: Oxford University Press.

US Committee on the Judiciary, House of Representatives (1996) *The Growing Threat of International Organized Crime: Hearing before the Subcommittee on Crime,* second session, 25 January, Serial No. 83, Washington DC: US Government Printing Office.

Wilson, J. Q. (1985) *Thinking about Crime* (2nd edition), New York: Vintage Books.

Zimring, F. E. and Hawkins, G. (1997) *The Search for Rational Drug Control,* Cambridge: Cambridge University Press.

Index

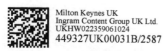

Milton Keynes UK
Ingram Content Group UK Ltd.
UKHW022359061024
449327UK00031B/2587

9 780415 192613